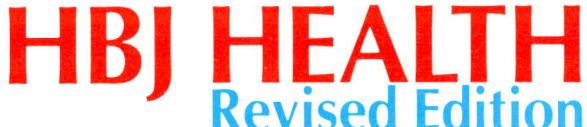

Red

Consulting Health Educators

Molly Kay Berger, R.N.
School Nurse/Health Educator
Fort Bend Independent School District
Sugarland, Texas

Barbara A. Galpin
Teacher of Health and Physical
* Education*
Islip Public Schools
Islip, New York

Kathleen Middleton
Director
National Center for Health Education
Concord, California

Linda Monroe
Classroom Teacher
Eustis Heights Elementary School
Eustis, Florida

Judith K. Scheer
Formerly Associate Professor
Department of Health Education
The University of Toledo
Toledo, Ohio

Joel B. Shapiro
Teacher of Elementary School Health
* and Physical Education*
Community School District 10
Bronx, New York

Debby Yeates
Classroom Teacher
Forest Hills Elementary School
Florence, Alabama

Nancy L. Young
Classroom Teacher and Supervisor of
* Student Teachers*
Royerton Elementary School
Muncie, Indiana

Consulting Health Specialists

Barbara L. Flye, Ph.D.
Director of Clinical Services
Andrus Home for Children
Yonkers, New York

Janice Gilyard-Robinson, R.N.
Assistant Professor and
* Pediatric Nurse Specialist*
School of Nursing
The University of North Carolina
* at Greensboro*

Wesley Halpert, D.D.S.
Clinical Professor of Dentistry
Columbia University School of Dental
* and Oral Surgery*
New York, New York

Irwin Rappaport, M.D., F.A.A.P.
Clinical Associate Professor of Pediatrics
Director, Allergy and Immunology
Department of Pediatrics
The New York Hospital
Cornell University Medical Center
New York, New York

Consulting Reading Specialists

Marjorie Slavick Frank
Specialist in Reading and
* Language Development*
Brooklyn, New York

P. J. Hutchins
Supervisor
Bureau of Reading Education
New York State Education Department
New York, New York

HBJ HARCOURT BRACE JOVANOVICH, PUBLISHERS
Orlando San Diego Chicago Dallas

Copyright © 1987 by Harcourt Brace Jovanovich, Inc.
All rights reserved. No part of this publication may be
reproduced or transmitted in any form or by any means,
electronic or mechanical, including photocopy, recording,
or any information storage and retrieval system, without
permission in writing from the publisher.

Requests for permission to make copies of any part of the work
should be mailed to: Permissions, Harcourt Brace Jovanovich,
Publishers, Orlando, Florida 32887

Material from earlier editions: copyright © 1983 by Harcourt Brace
Jovanovich, Inc. All rights reserved.

Printed in the United States of America

ISBN 0-15-369002-X

PHOTOGRAPH ACKNOWLEDGMENTS
COVER: Richard Hutchings.
Key: t(top), b(bottom), c(center), l(left), r(right).
2, Susan McCartney/Photo Researchers, Inc.; 3, Susan McCartney/Photo Researchers, Inc.; 4, HBJ Photo/Ken Lax; 5, HBJ Photo/Ken Lax; 6, HBJ Photo/Rosmarie Hausherr; 7, HBJ Photo/Rosmarie Hausherr; 8, HBJ Photo/Ken Lax; 9, HBJ Photo/Rosmarie Hausherr; 10, Bob Martin; 12, HBJ Photo/Rosmarie Hausherr; 13, HBJ Photo/Rosmarie Hausherr; 14, HBJ Photo/Ken Lax; 15, HBJ Photo/Rosmarie Hausherr; 16, HBJ Photo/Ken Lax; 17, HBJ Photo/Ken Lax; 18, HBJ Photo/Rosmarie Hausherr; 22, HBJ Photo/Rosmarie Hausherr; 23, HBJ Photo/Rosmarie Hausherr; 24, Four by Five; 25, Bob Bendick/Monkmeyer Press Photo Service; 26, HBJ Photo/Ken Lax; 27, HBJ Photo/Ken Lax; 28(l), HBJ Photo/Ken Lax; 28(r), Guy Gillette/Photo Researchers, Inc.; 29(l), Dunn/DPI; 29(r), John G. O'Connor/Monkmeyer Press Photo Service; 30(bl), HBJ Photo/Rosmarie Hausherr; 30(bl), HBJ Photo/Ken Lax; 30(cl), Shostal Associates; 30(r), HBJ Photo/Rosmarie Hausherr; 30(tl), HBJ Photo/Ken Lax; 34, HBJ Photo/Rosmarie Hausherr; 36, H. Armstrong Roberts; 37, HBJ Photo/Rosmarie Hausherr; 38, HBJ Photo/Rosmarie Hausherr; 39, HBJ Photo/Rosmarie Hausherr; 40, Richard Steedman/The Image Bank; 44, HBJ Photo/Ken Lax; 45, HBJ Photo/Ken Lax; 46, HBJ Photo/James Gilmour; 47, HBJ Photo/James Gilmour; 48, HBJ Photo/James Gilmour; 49, HBJ Photo/James Gilmour; 50, HBJ Photo/James Gilmour; 51, HBJ Photo/James Gilmour; 52, HBJ Photo/James Gilmour; 53, HBJ Photo/James Gilmour; 54(bl), Shostal Associates; 54(r), HBJ Photo/Rosmarie Hausherr; 54(tl), Shostal Associates; 55, HBJ Photo/James Gilmour; 58, HBJ Photo/Rosmarie Hausherr; 59, HBJ Photo/James Gilmour; 60, HBJ Photo/James Gilmour; 61, HBJ Photo/Rosmarie Hausherr; 66, HBJ Photo/Rosmarie Hausherr; 67, HBJ Photo/Rosmarie Hausherr; 72, HBJ Photo/Rosmarie Hausherr; 73, HBJ Photo/Ken Lax; 76(l), Glenn H. Baer/Shostal Associates; 76(r), HBJ Photo/Ken Lax; 77, HBJ Photo/Ken Lax; 78, HBJ Photo/Rosmarie Hausherr; 79(bl), Jeffrey E. Blackman/Vista Photography, Inc.; 79(r), Jeffrey E. Blackman/Vista Photography, Inc.; 79(tl), HBJ Photo/Ken Lax; 80, HBJ Photo/Rosmarie Hausherr; 84, HBJ Photo/Ken Lax; 85, HBJ Photo/Ken Lax; 86, David York/Medichrome (A Division of The Stock Shop, Inc.); 87(br), HBJ Photo/James Gilmour; 87(l), Eric Grave/Phototake; 87(tr), HBJ Photo/James Gilmour; 88, HBJ Photo/Ken Lax; 89, HBJ Photo/Rosmarie Hausherr; 90, HBJ Photo/Ken Lax; 91, HBJ Photo/Ken Lax; 92, HBJ Photo/Rosmarie Hausherr; 93, HBJ Photo/Rosmarie Hausherr; 94, HBJ Photo/Ken Lax; 95, HBJ Photo/Ken Lax; 96, HBJ Photo/Ken Lax; 97, HBJ Photo/James Gilmour; 98, Smith-Kettlewell Institute of Visual Sciences; 100, HBJ Photo/Ken Lax; 101, HBJ Photo/Ken Lax; 102, HBJ Photo/Ken Lax; 103, HBJ Photo/Ken Lax; 104, HBJ Photo/Ken Lax; 108, HBJ Photo/Ken Lax; 109, HBJ Photo/Ken Lax; 110, HBJ Photo/Ken Lax; 111, HBJ Photo/Rosmarie Hausherr; 112, HBJ Photo/James Gilmour; 113, HBJ Photo/James Gilmour; 116, HBJ Photo/Ken Lax; 117, HBJ Photo/Ken Lax; 118, HBJ Photo/James Gilmour; 119, HBJ Photo/Ken Lax; 120, HBJ Photo/Ken Lax; 121, HBJ Photo/Ken Lax; 122, HBJ Photo/James Gilmour; 124, HBJ Photo/James Gilmour; 125, HBJ Photo/James Gilmour; 130, HBJ Photo/Rosmarie Hausherr; 131, HBJ Photo/Ken Lax; 132, HBJ Photo/Rosmarie Hausherr; 133, HBJ Photo/Rosmarie Hausherr; 134, HBJ Photo/Ken Lax; 135, HBJ Photo/Ken Lax; 138, HBJ Photo/Ken Lax; 139, HBJ Photo/Rosmarie Hausherr; 140, HBJ Photo/Ken Lax; 141, HBJ Photo/Ken Lax; 142, HBJ Photo/Ken Lax; 143, Eric Carle/Shostal Associates; 144, HBJ Photo/Rosmarie Hausherr; 145, HBJ Photo/Rosmarie Hausherr; 146, HBJ Photo/Rosmarie Hausherr; 147, HBJ Photo/Ken Lax; 148, HBJ Photo/Ken Lax; 152, HBJ Photo/Rosmarie Hausherr; 153, HBJ Photo/Rosmarie Hausherr; 154, HBJ Photo/Ken Lax; 155, HBJ Photo/Ken Lax; 156, HBJ Photo/Ken Lax; 157, HBJ Photo/Ken Lax; 158, HBJ Photo/James Gilmour; 159, HBJ Photo/Rosmarie Hausherr; 160, HBJ Photo/James Gilmour; 161, HBJ Photo/Rosmarie Hausherr; 162, Jean Tinguely, Fragment from Homage to New York (1960) Painted metal, 6' 8-1/2" x 29-5/8" x 7' 3-7/8"; 164, Tom Tracy/The Stock Shop; 165, HBJ Photo/Ken Lax; 166, HBJ Photo/Ken Lax; 167, HBJ Photo/Ken Lax; 168, HBJ Photo/Ken Lax; 169, HBJ Photo/Ken Lax; 170, HBJ Photo/Ken Lax; 174, HBJ Photo/Rosmarie Hausherr; 175, HBJ Photo/Rosmarie Hausherr; 176, HBJ Photo/Ken Lax; 177, HBJ Photo/Rosmarie Hausherr; 178, HBJ Photo/Rosmarie Hausherr; 179, HBJ Photo/Rosmarie Hausherr.

ART ACKNOWLEDGMENTS
Teresa Anderko: 19, 81, 171. Doran Ben-Ami: 32. Susan Blubaugh: 56, 62, 114. Carol Ann Morley: 31, 35, 41, 68, 69, 70, 71, 123. Heidi Palmer: 126, 127, 149. Marti Shohet: 74, 105. Jerry Smath: 11, 33, 57, 63, 75, 99, 115, 136, 137, 163, all "Do You Remember" chalk boards, and all "Health Check-Up" toucans.

CONTENTS

1 Everyone Has Feelings   2

Understanding Feelings   4
Feelings Can Change   6
Feelings Can Show   8
Health Highlight: A Story Without Words   10
Going, Seeing, and Doing   11
Getting Along with Others   12
A Family Cares and Shares   14
A Family Works Together   16
Your Turn: A Hard Day   18
Health in Action   19
Do You Remember?   20
Health Check-Up   21

2 Growing Inside and Out   22

Everyone Is Different   24
You Grow in Many Ways   26
Growing Isn't Just Getting Bigger   28
Your Eyes and Ears Help You Grow   30
Health Highlight: Seeing Colors Differently   32
Going, Seeing, and Doing   33
Other Senses Help You Grow   34
Health Habits for Growing   36
More Habits for Growing   38

iii

Your Turn: Learning and Growing   40
Health in Action   41
Do You Remember?   42
Health Check-Up   43

3 Choosing Your Foods   44

Different Foods   46
Foods for Health—The Fruit and Vegetable Group   48
Foods for Health—The Meat Group   50
Foods for Health—The Milk Group   52
Foods for Health—The Bread and Cereal Group   54
Health Highlight: Krill for Lunch   56
Going, Seeing, and Doing   57
Healthful Meals   58
Snacks and Your Health   60
Your Turn: At the Restaurant   62
Health in Action   63
Do You Remember?   64
Health Check-Up   65

4 Your Teeth   66

Teeth You Lose and Teeth You Keep   68
Parts of a Tooth   70
Taking Care of Your Teeth   72
Health Highlight: A Toothbrush Is Born   74
Going, Seeing, and Doing   75

Getting Help for Your Teeth 76
Protecting Your Teeth from Injury 78
Your Turn: No Toothbrush 80
Health in Action 81
Do You Remember? 82
Health Check-Up 83

5 Taking Care of Your Health 84

Knowing About Germs 86
Germs Can Spread 88
Sometimes You May Feel Ill 90
A Cold Is Not Something to Share 92
The Doctor Looks 94
Wearing Glasses 96
Health Highlight: A Machine that Sees and Talks 98
Going, Seeing, and Doing 99
The Doctor Listens 100
Following Good Advice 102
Your Turn: Fuzzy Words 104
Health in Action 105
Do You Remember? 106
Health Check-Up 107

6 Knowing About Drugs 108

Sometimes Medicine Can Help 110
First, Read the Label 112

v

Health Highlight: Medicine from Nature   114
Going, Seeing, and Doing   115
Your Own Medicine   116
Poisons   118
Asking for Help   120
Smoking Isn't Healthy   122
Caffeine Isn't Healthy   124
Your Turn: Making a Healthful Choice   126
Health in Action   127
Do You Remember?   128
Health Check-Up   129

7 Safety in Your World   130

Cars, Corners, and Crosswalks   132
Riding Bicycles   134
Health Highlight: The First Bicycle Tires   136
Going, Seeing, and Doing   137
Riding in Buses and Cars   138
Being Careful Around Animals   140
Safety Outside   142
Safety Inside   144
When Accidents Happen   146
Your Turn: A Stray Dog   148
Health in Action   149
Do You Remember?   150
Health Check-Up   151

8 The World Around You   152

Helping Your World   154
Saving Energy   156
Saving Paper and Water   158
Using Things Again   160
Health Highlight: Junk Art   162
Going, Seeing, and Doing   163
The Noise Around You   164
Helping to Care for the Outdoors   166
Helping to Care for Your Home   168
Your Turn: The Gift Box   170
Health in Action   171
Do You Remember?   172
Health Check-Up   173

Exercise Handbook   174
Reviewing the Health Words   180
Index   183

CHAPTER 1

Everyone Has Feelings

You have feelings. So does everyone else. Knowing about feelings is important. It can help you understand yourself and others. It can help you get along with others, too.

Why is it important to get along with others?

Health Words

happy	thoughtful
sad	love
feelings	share
afraid	family members

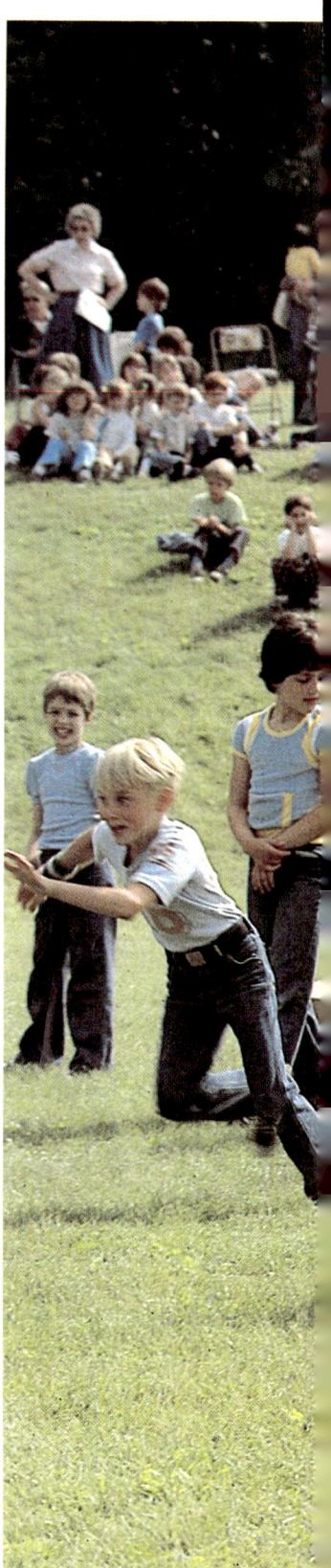

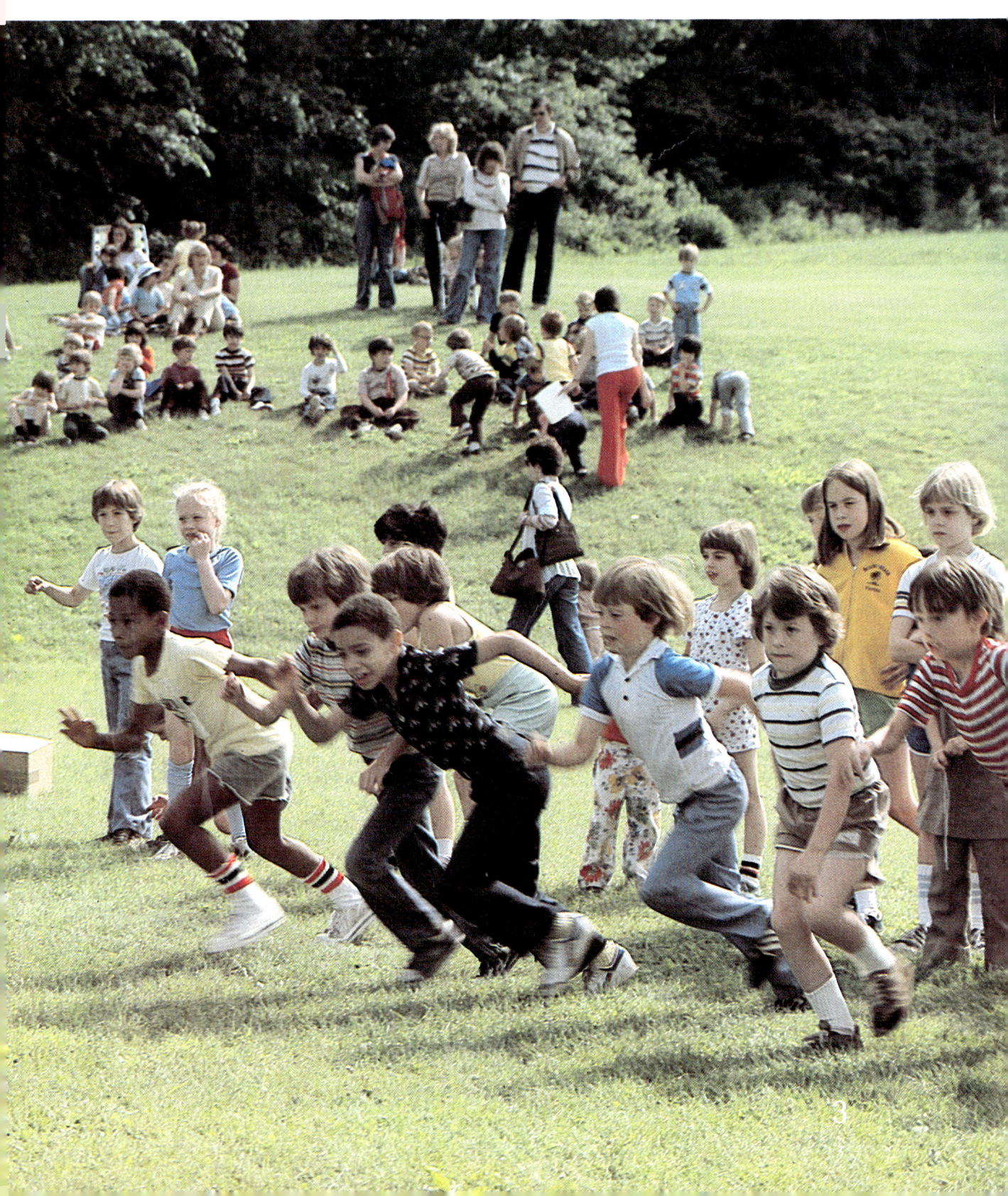

Understanding Your Feelings

You have many different feelings. Some things may make you happy. Other things may make you sad or angry or afraid.

All your feelings are important. They are important because they are part of you.

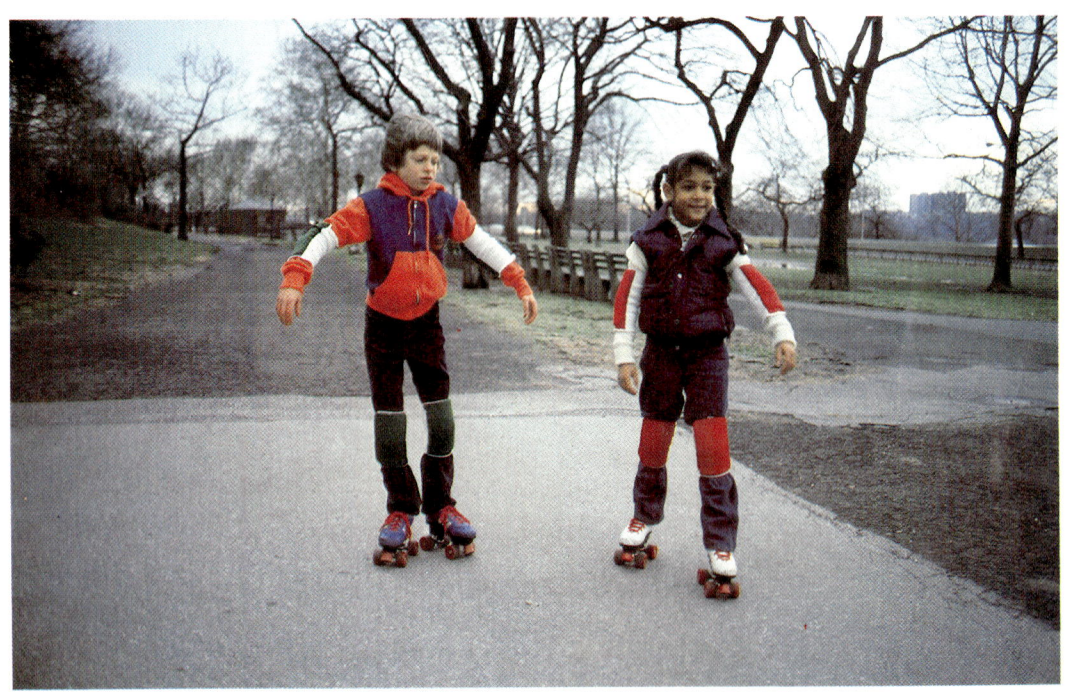

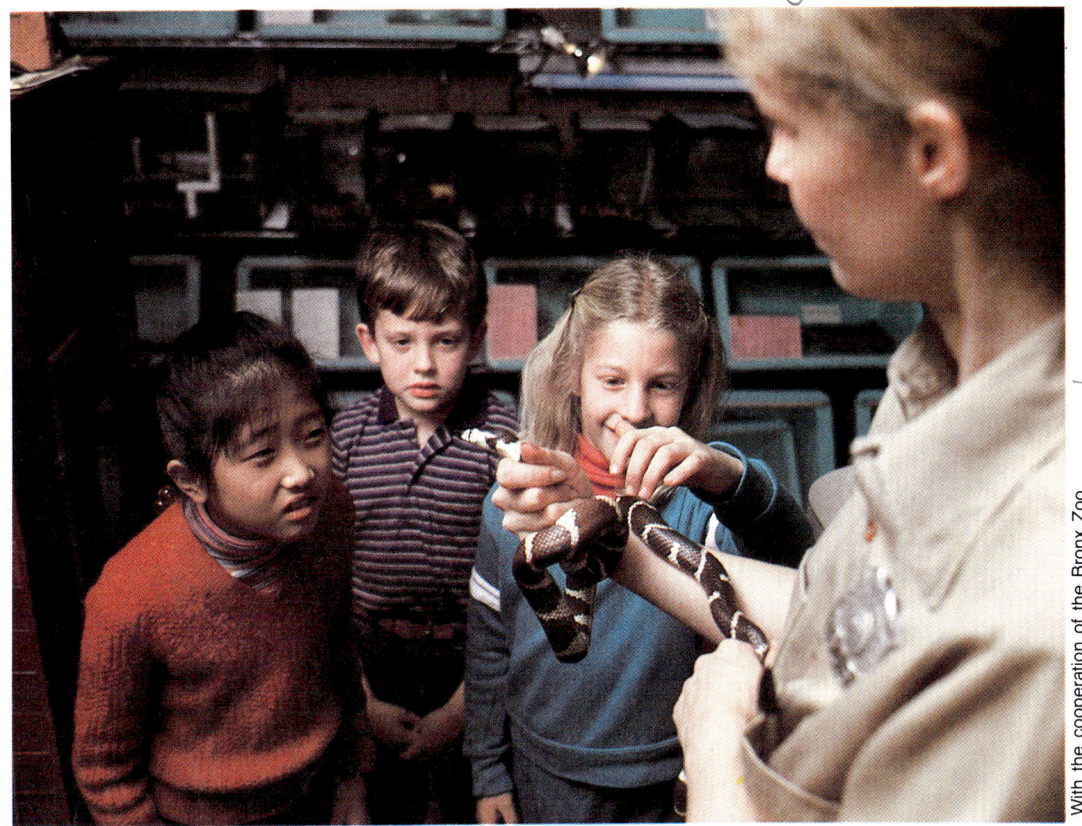

Look at the picture on page 4.
Tell how the children feel.
Tell why they might feel that way.

Look at the picture on this page.
How does each child feel?
Tell how you would feel.
Why is it important to understand your feelings?

Feelings Can Change

Your feelings can change. There are times when you may feel happy about something. At other times, that same thing may make you feel sad or angry.

Others have feelings, too. Their feelings may be different from yours, but they are just as important as yours.

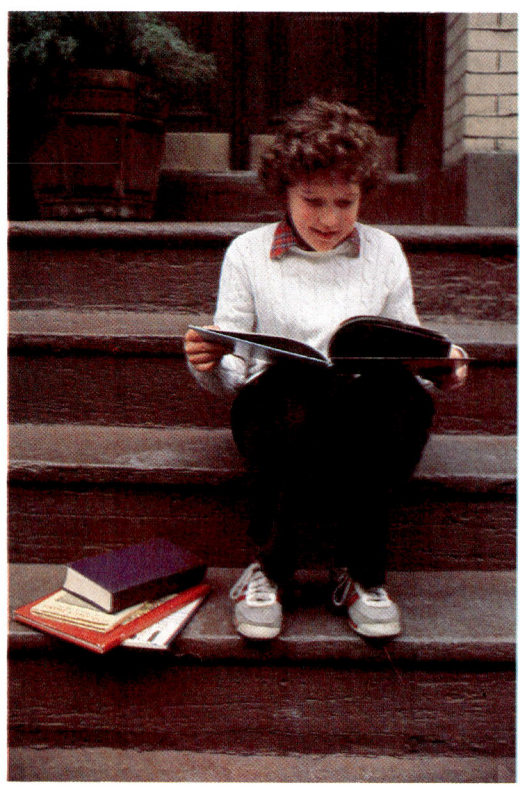 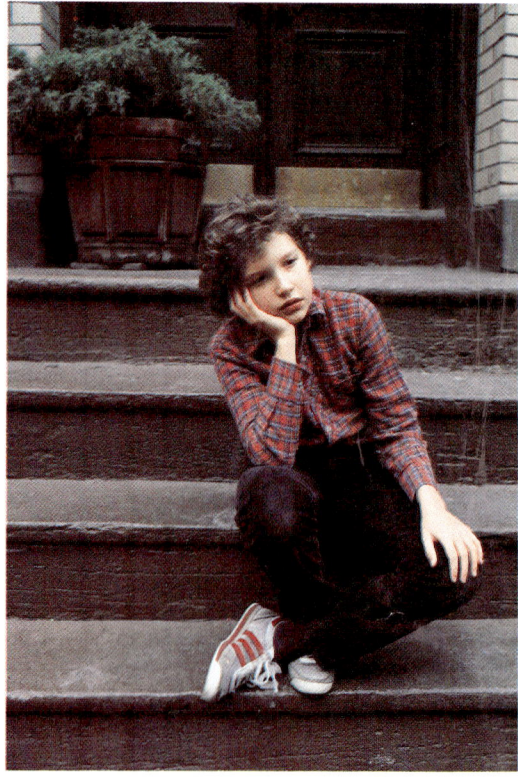

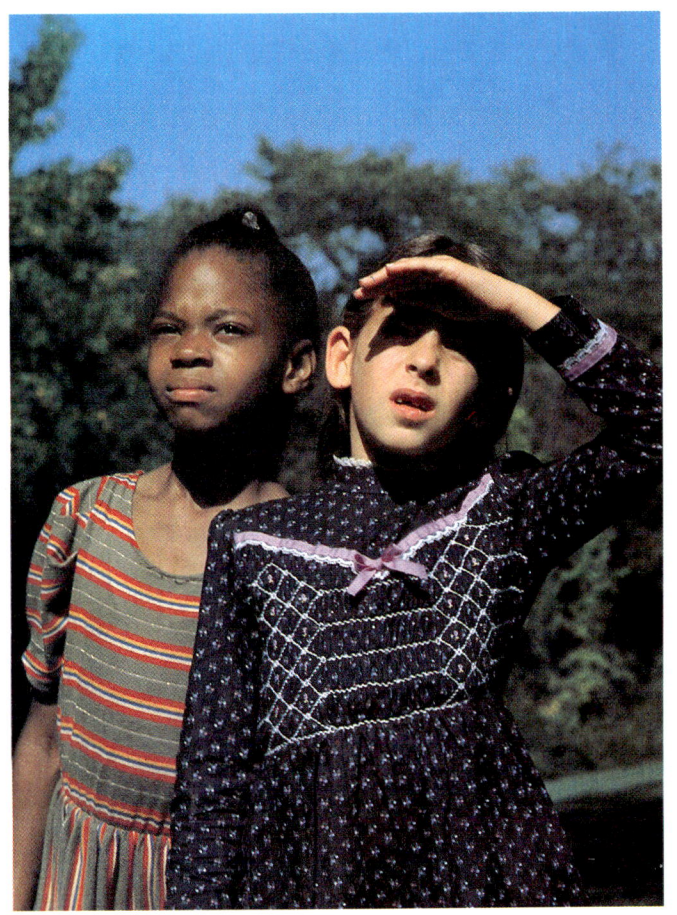 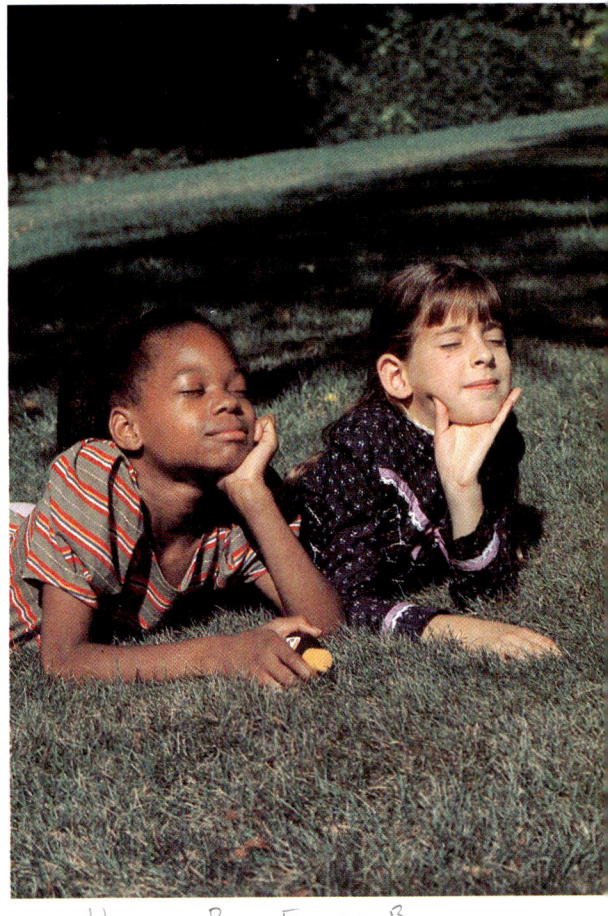

Look at the pictures on page 6.

How does the boy feel in each picture?

Look at the girls on this page.
Tell how their feelings change.
Tell about other times when the sun might make someone happy.

Feelings Can Show

There are many ways to show your feelings. You can show them by what you do or say. You can show them in your face, too. You may smile or you may frown. Tears may show that you're afraid or angry or sad.

Knowing when and how to show your feelings is part of being healthy.

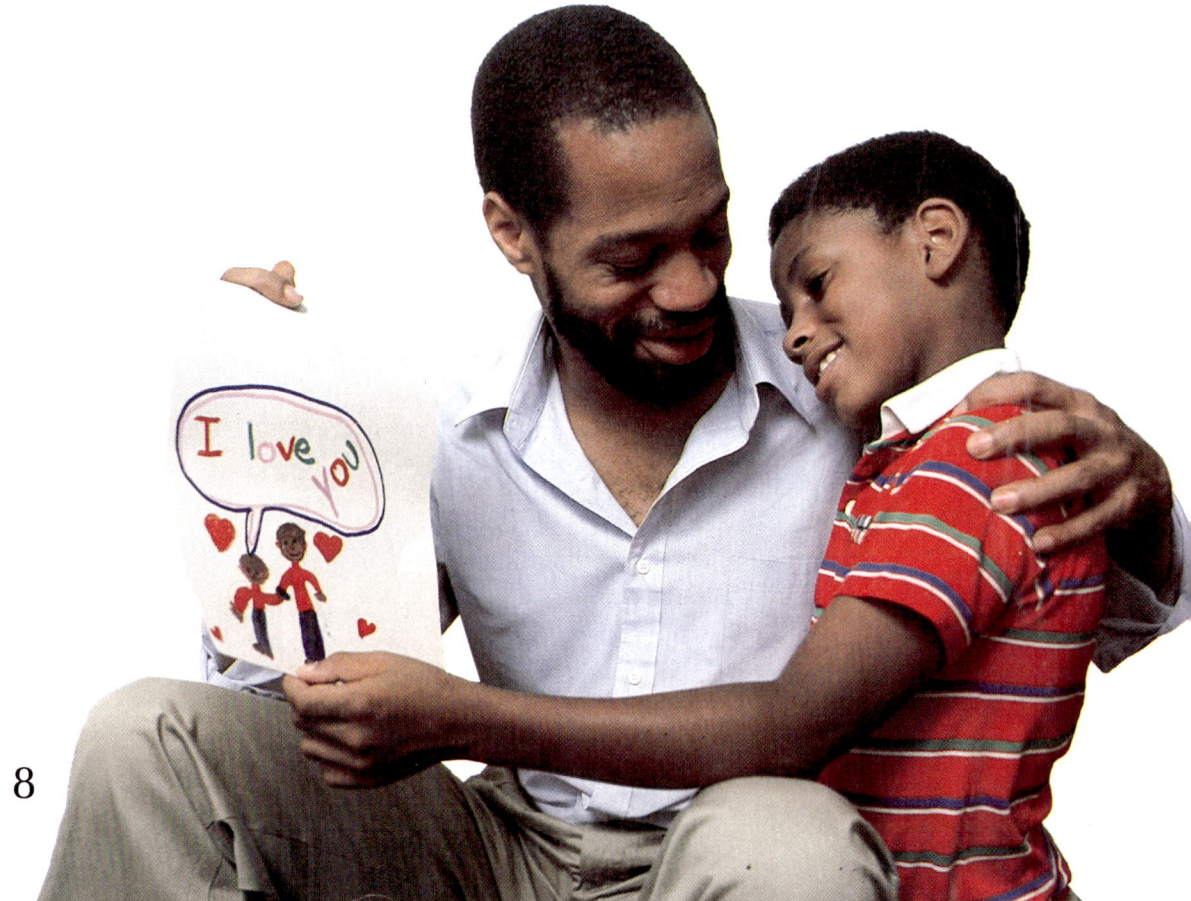

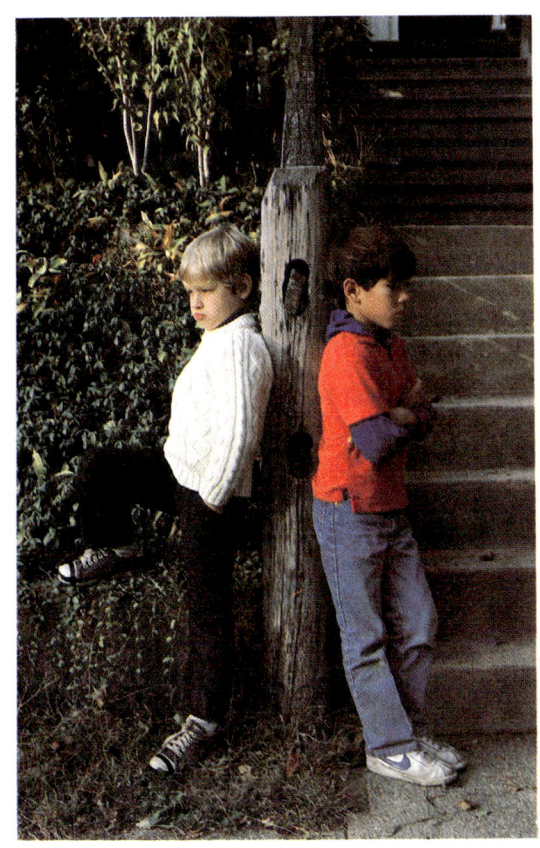
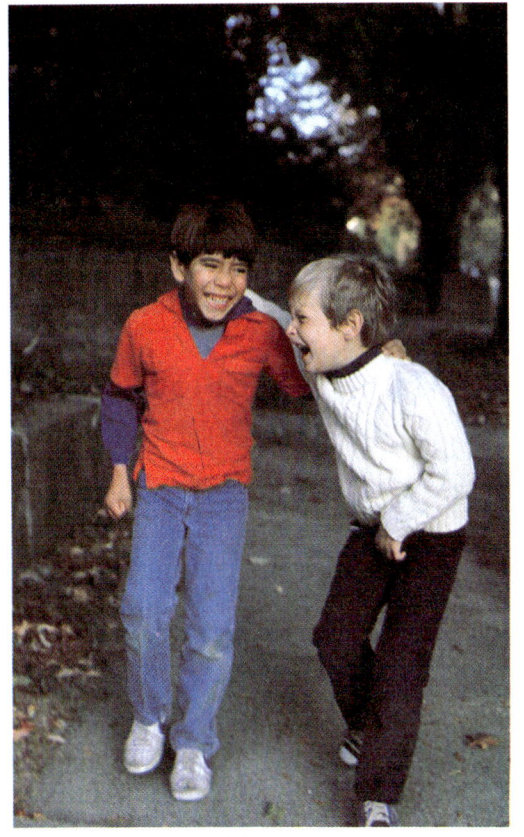

Look at the picture on page 8.
How does the boy feel about the grown-up?
How is he showing his feelings?
Show this feeling in another way.

Look at each picture on this page.
Tell how the children feel.
How do you know?
Tell a way to make up with a friend.

Health Highlight

A Story Without Words

This man's name is Marcel Marceau. Mr. Marceau is a mime artist. He tells stories, but he doesn't talk. He acts out his stories. He uses his body and face. He shows what people do. He shows how they feel.

What feeling is Marcel Marceau showing now?

Tell some ways you talk without words.

Show a way.

Going, Seeing, and Doing

1. Find a quiet place. Sit down. Close your eyes. Keep them closed for one minute. Don't talk. Later, tell how you felt.

2. Watch the people around you. Look at their faces. Look at the things they are doing. Try to guess how some of the people are feeling.

3. Make believe you are at a picnic. It has just started to rain. Tell how you would feel. Now, pretend your garden needs water. Show your feelings about rain.

Getting Along with Others

Getting along with others can be easy. Think of how you would like others to treat you. Treat them the same way. Share when you can. Be thoughtful. Listen to what they say. Try to understand how they feel.

Getting along with others can help you feel good about yourself. It can help others feel good, too.

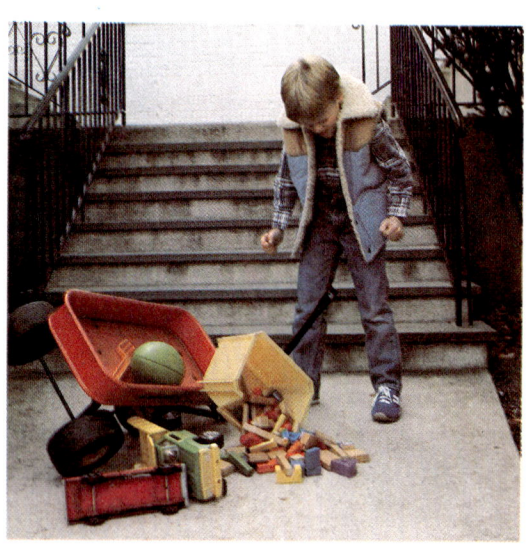
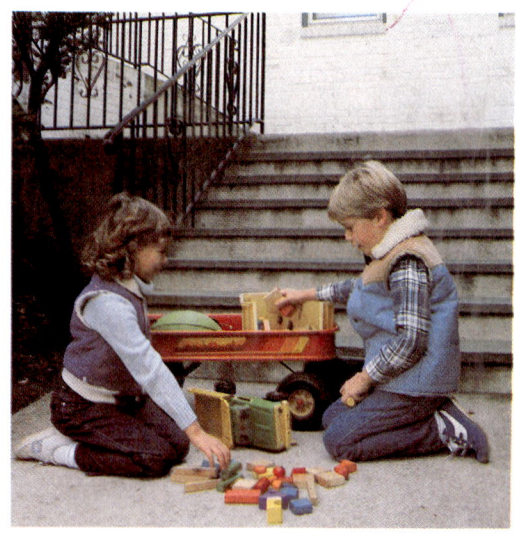

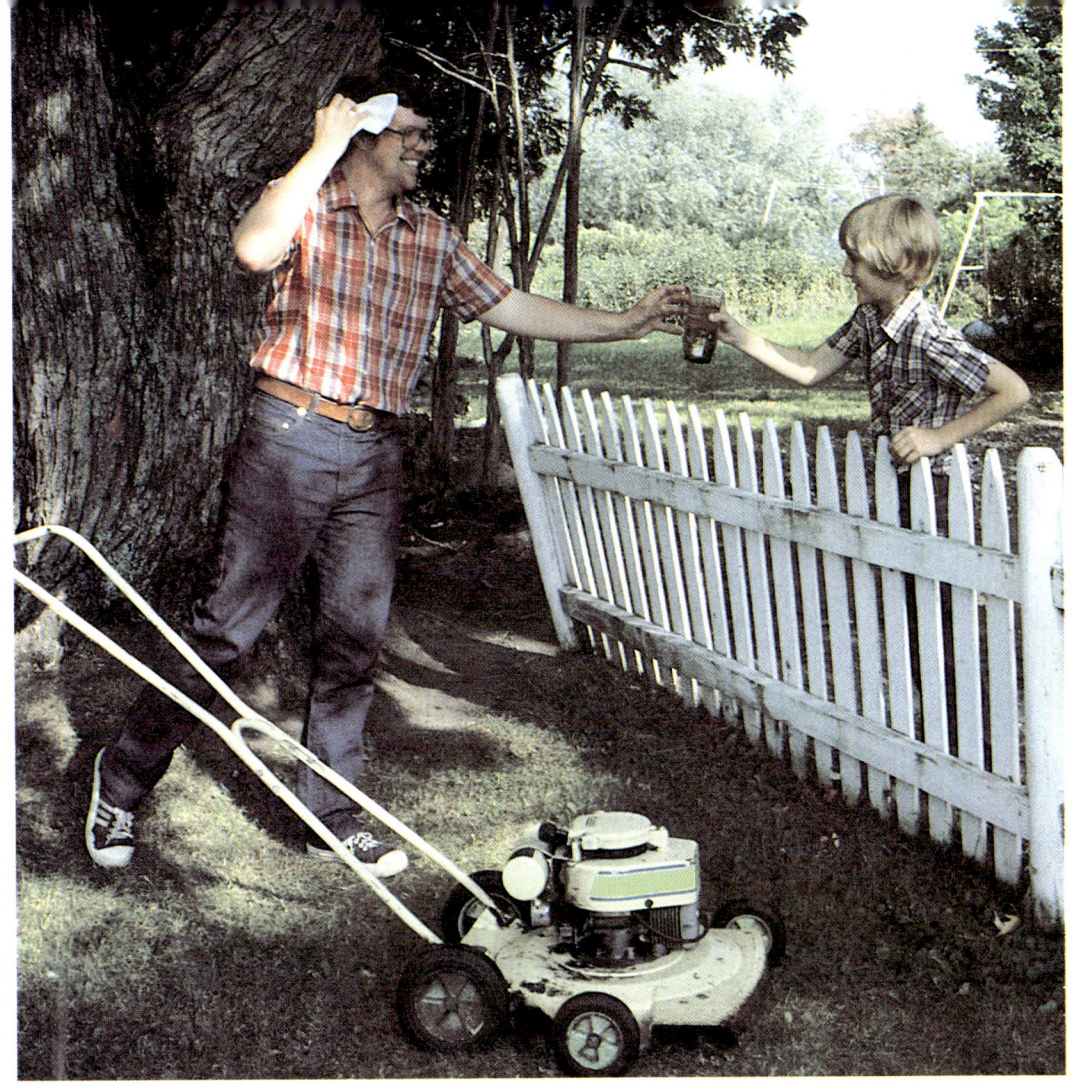

Look at the pictures on page 12.

Who is being thoughtful?

How is that person being thoughtful?

How did being thoughtful help?

Look at the picture on this page.

Tell how the boy helped.

How else can you help others?

A Family Cares and Shares

Family members can care about one another. They can watch out for one another. They can help and love one another. They can listen and they can share. Everyone is part of a family. Every person in a family is special. Being special can feel very good.

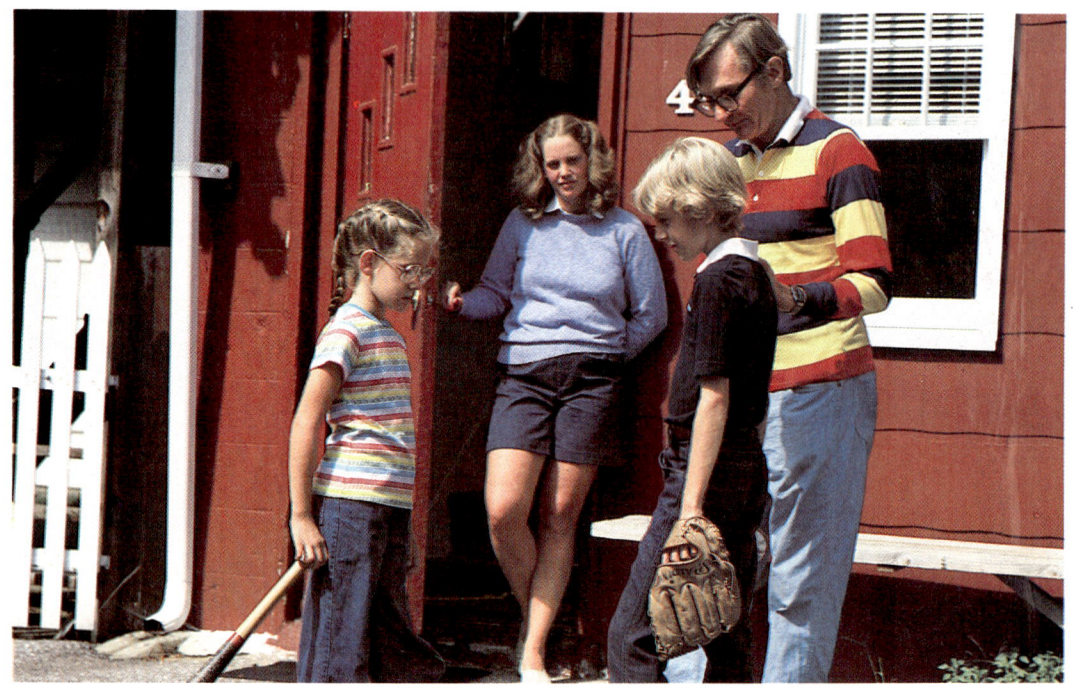

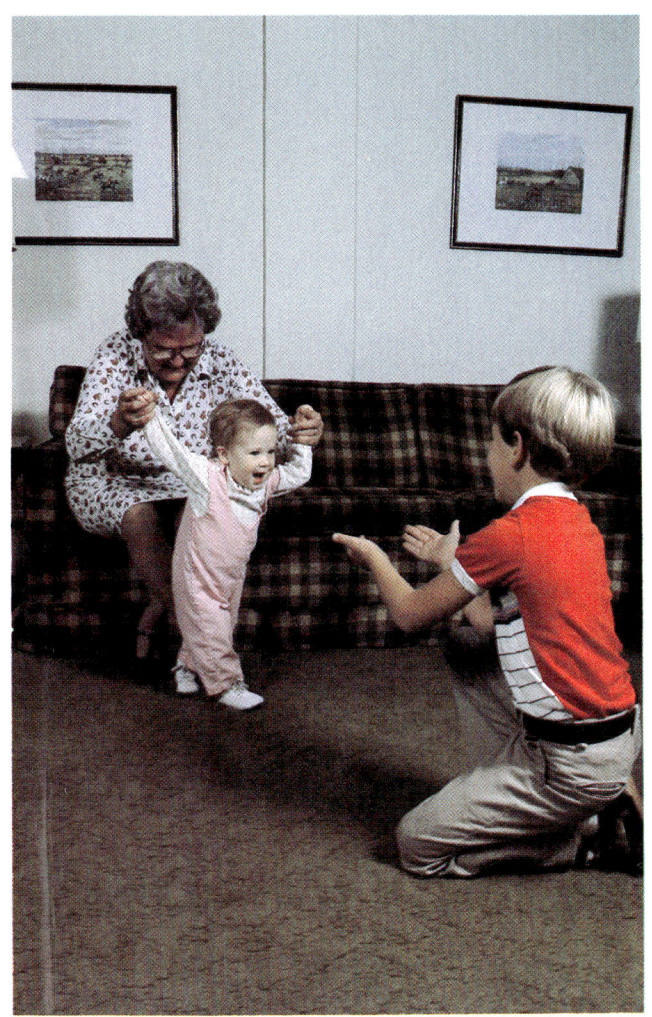
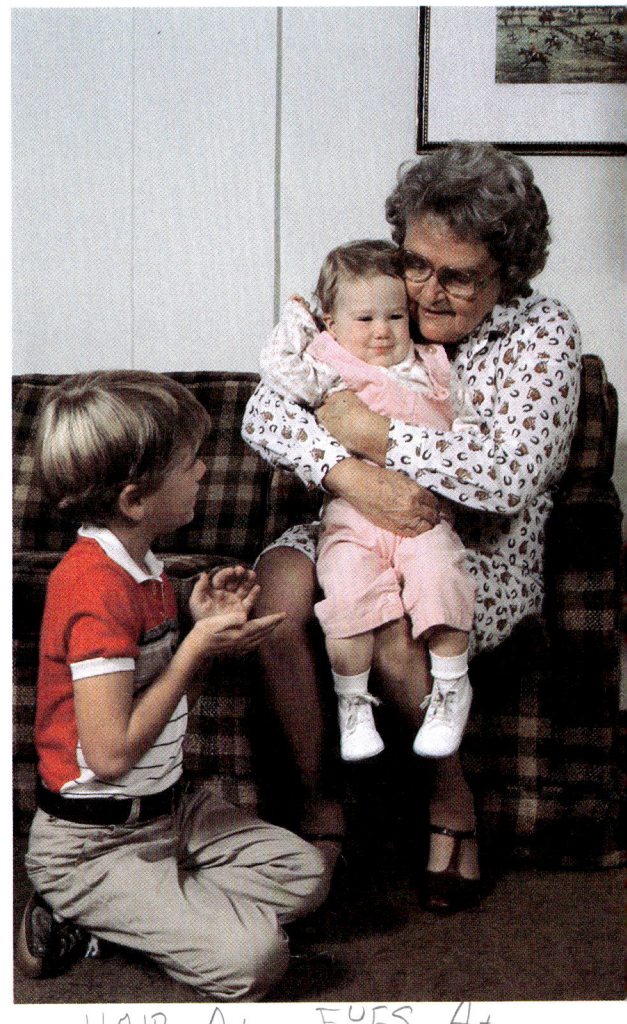

Look at all three pictures.

How do you know the family members love one another?

How else can family members show they care about one another?

Tell why family members are special.

15

A Family Works Together

There are many kinds of jobs to do at home, but there are many ways to get them done. Family members can work together. Everyone can share the work. Then, no one has to do everything. When family members work together, the whole family is better off.

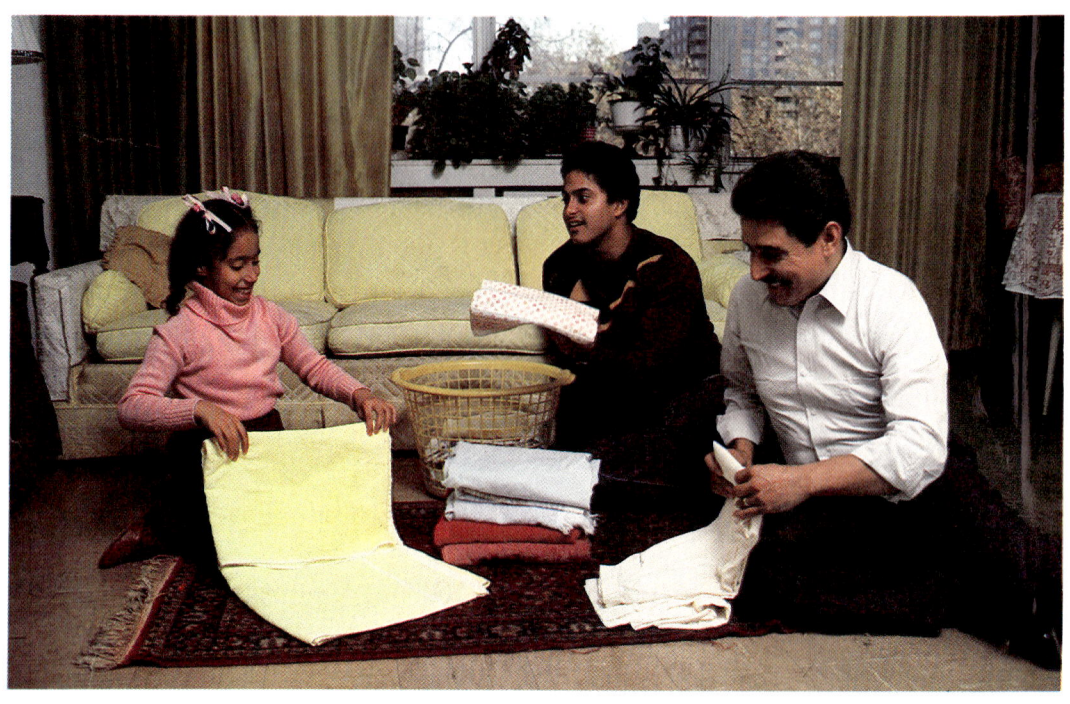

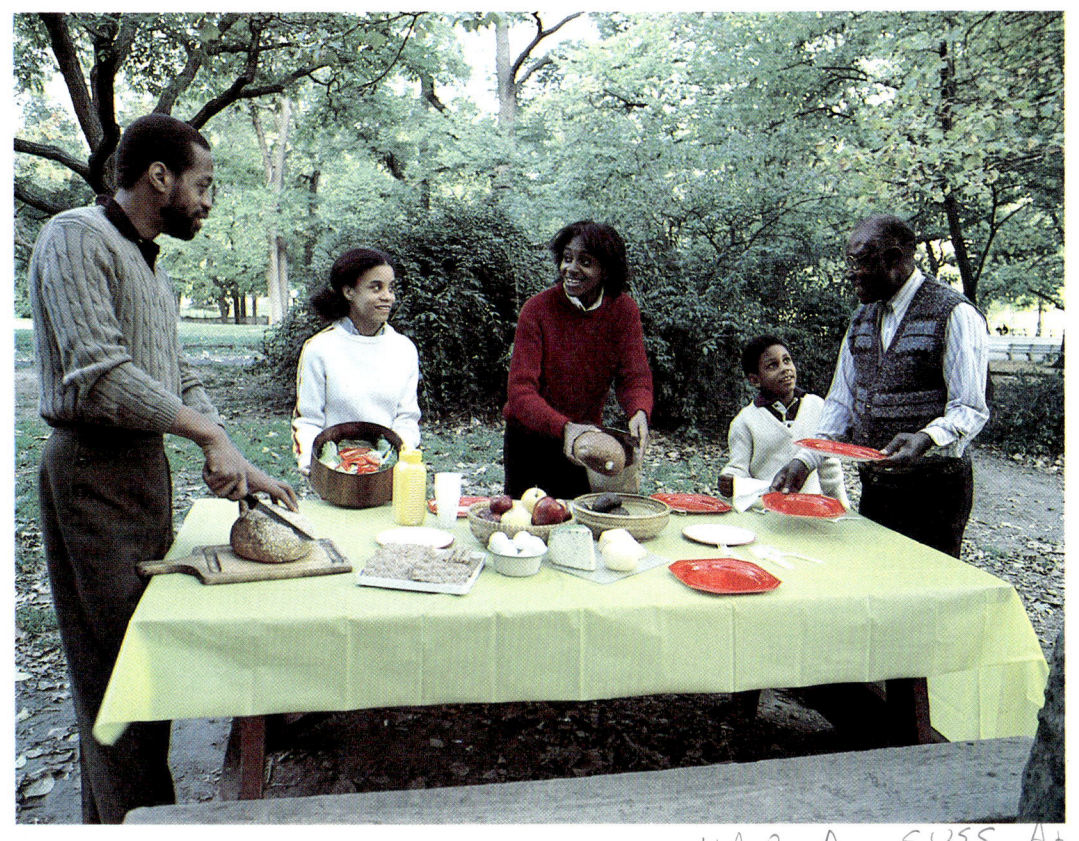

Look at both pictures.

Tell how the family members are working together.

How is each family member helping?

Why is each job important for the family's health?

Act out other family jobs.

Tell why they are important.

17

Your Turn

A Hard Day

Mr. Brooks is very tired. He worked hard all day. Then, he came home and cooked dinner for his family. Now he has more work to do. He has to clean up.

Make believe you are a member of the family.

Tell what you would do to help.
Tell why your ideas would help.

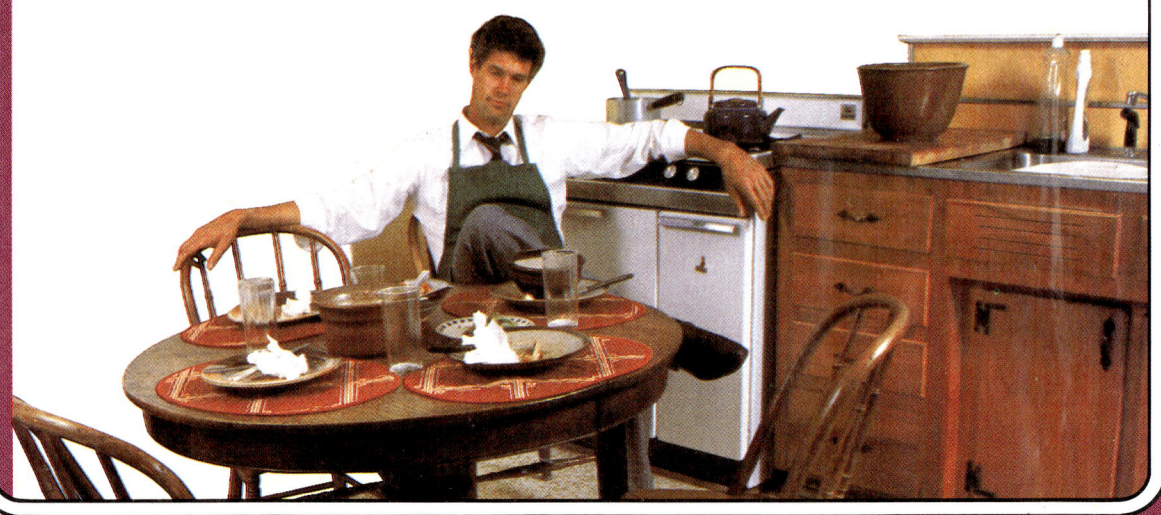

Health in Action

1. Look at the pictures. Tell how each makes you feel. Why do you feel that way?

2. Draw a picture. Show a way to be thoughtful. Then, tell about your picture.

3. Copy the list. Write a way to help in each room. Then, help in that way when you can.

   kitchen
   bedroom
   bathroom

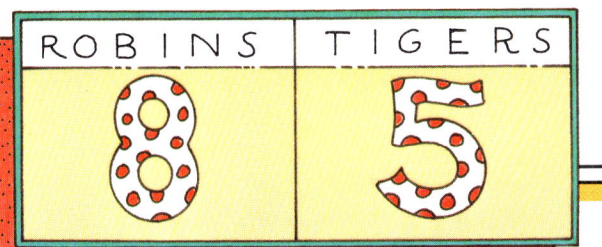

4. Write a news story. Tell who won the game. Tell the score. Tell how you think the members of each team may feel.

19

Do You Remember?

Your Health Words

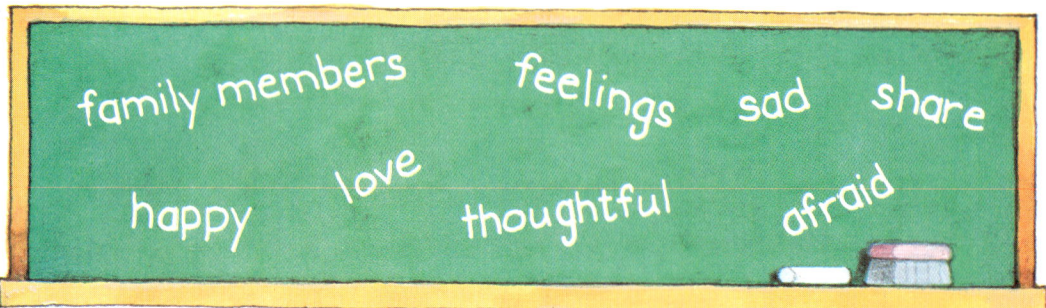

Finish the sentences.

Use the Health Words.

1. You can feel ___.
2. Brothers and sisters are ___.
3. You can be ___ of others.

Your Health Ideas

1. Show a feeling.
2. Tell some ways to get along with others.
3. Tell some ways family members can help one another.

Health Check-Up

Tell which sentences are true.

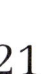

1. People have many kinds of feelings.
2. People always feel the same way about things.
3. Your feelings never change.
4. There are ways to show feelings.
5. It is important to know how to show feelings.
6. Sharing work can help you get along with others.
7. It is important to be thoughtful.
8. Family members cannot help one another.
9. All family members are special.
10. A family should work together.

CHAPTER 2

Growing Inside and Out

Something wonderful is happening. You are growing. You are not just growing bigger. You are growing up. You are learning to do new things. Learning is one way you grow. There are other ways, too.

What are some ways you grow?

Health Words

features	heart
growing	lungs
body	senses
muscle	energy

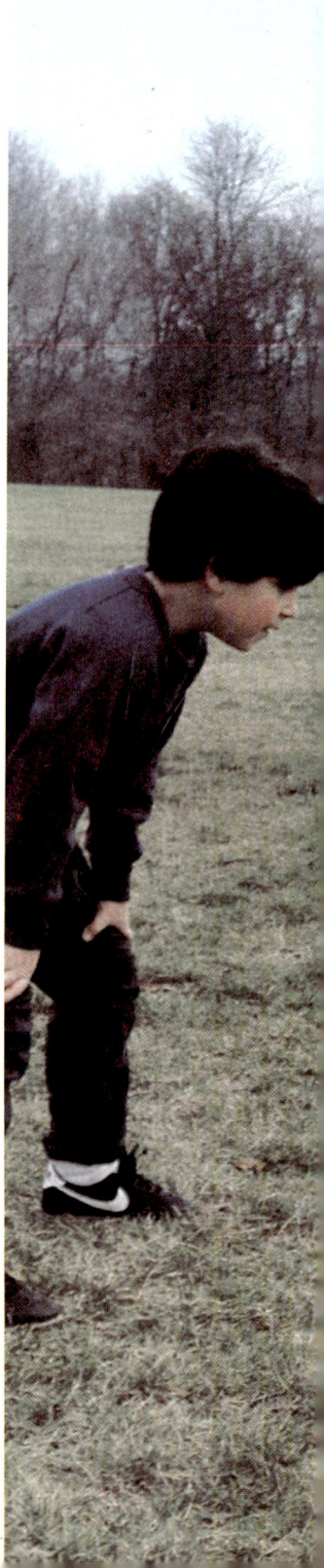

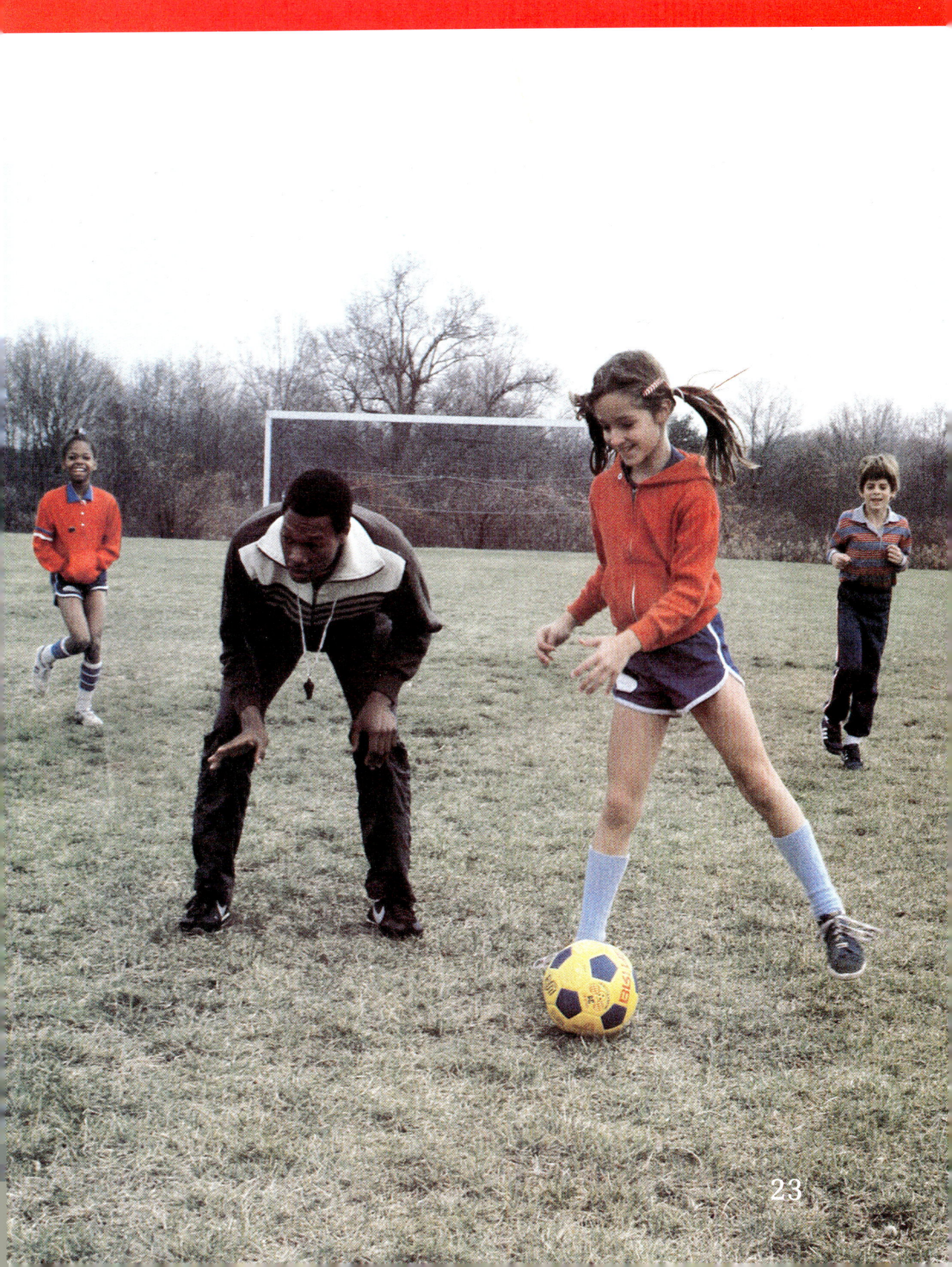

Everyone Is Different

You have your own special set of features. The color of your eyes is one feature. How tall you are is another. Family members may have some of your same features, but not all of them. Your features are very much your own. You are truly one of a kind.

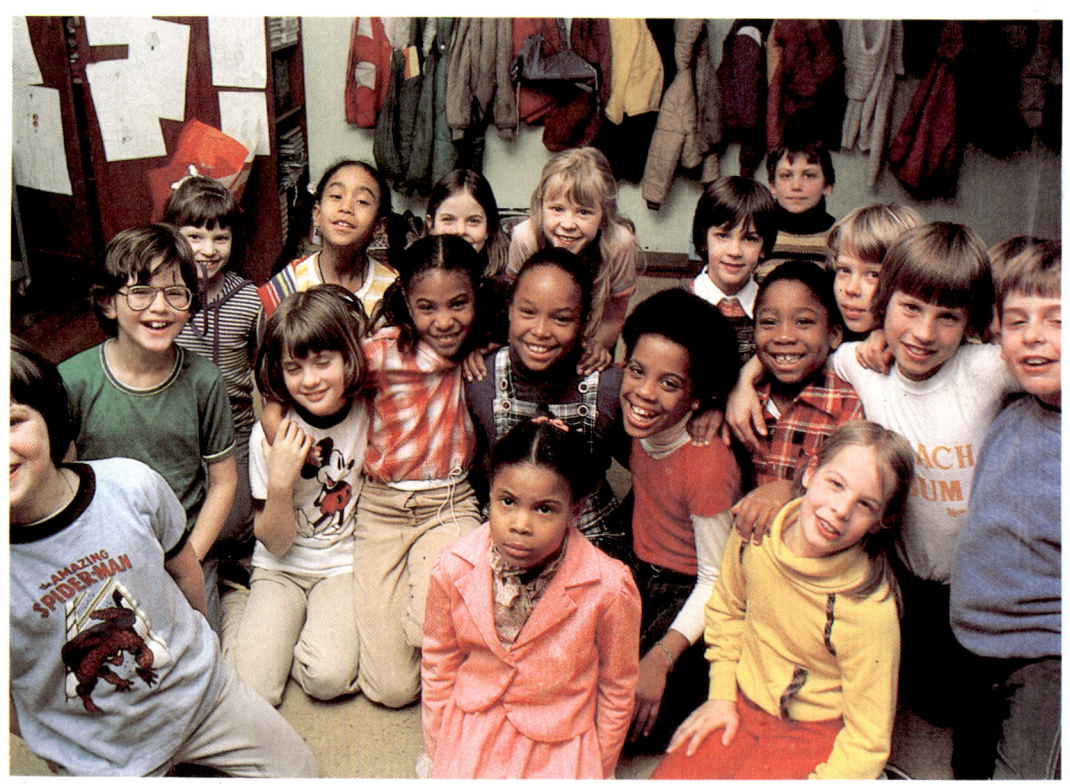

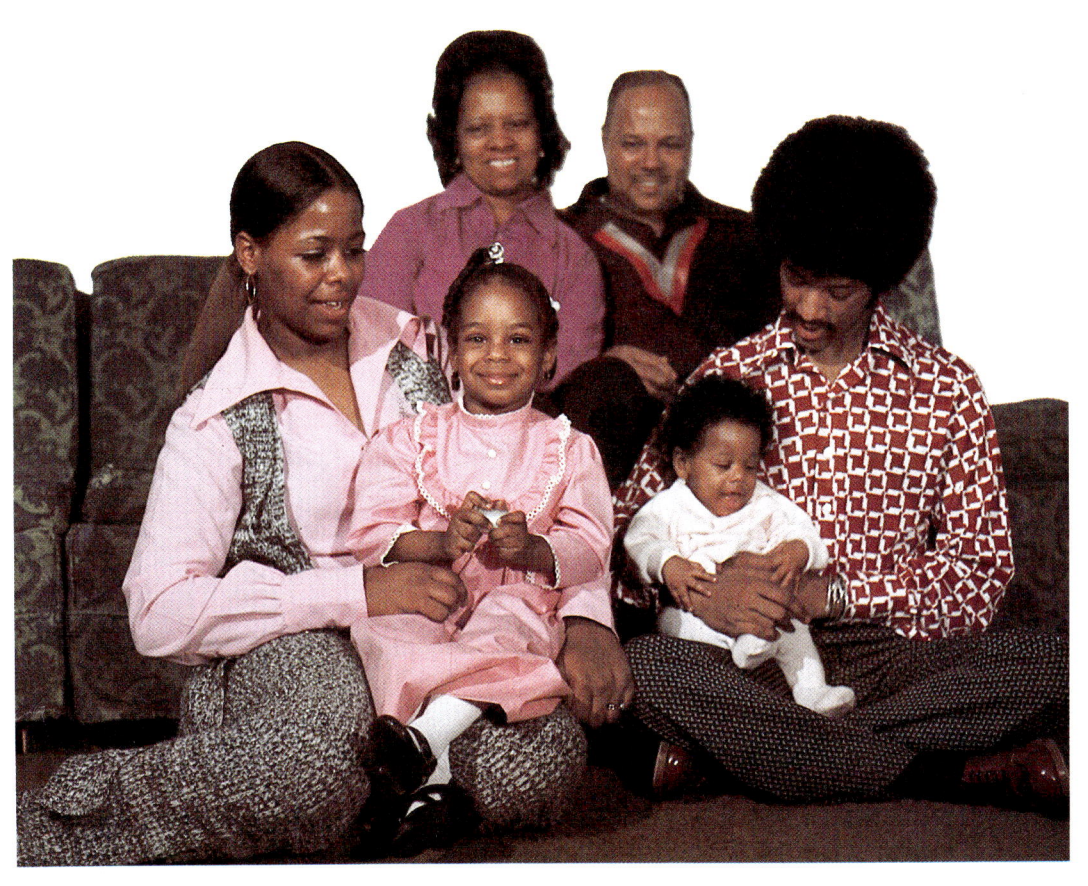

Look at the picture on page 24.

Tell how the children are different.

Look at the picture of the family.

In what ways do the family members look alike?

Tell some ways they are different.

Tell about your own features.

You Grow in Many Ways

Every part of your body is growing. Every bone. Every muscle. Even your heart and your lungs are growing.

You are growing in other ways, too. You are learning to do new things. Learning and growing are good for you. They are part of being healthy.

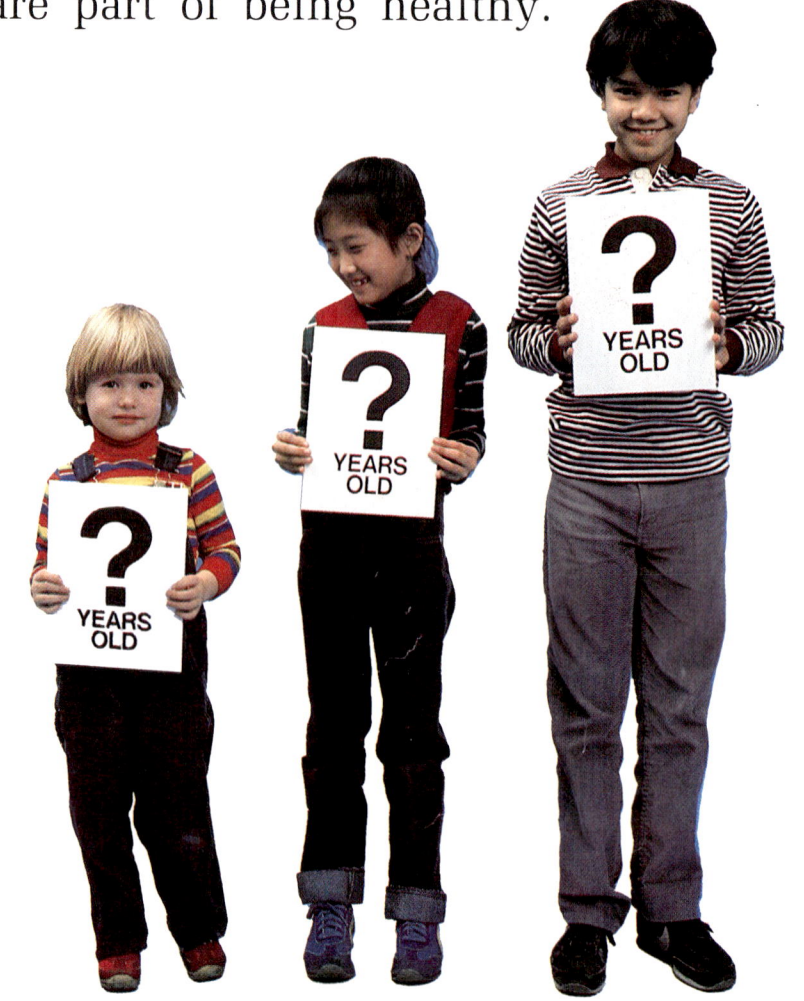

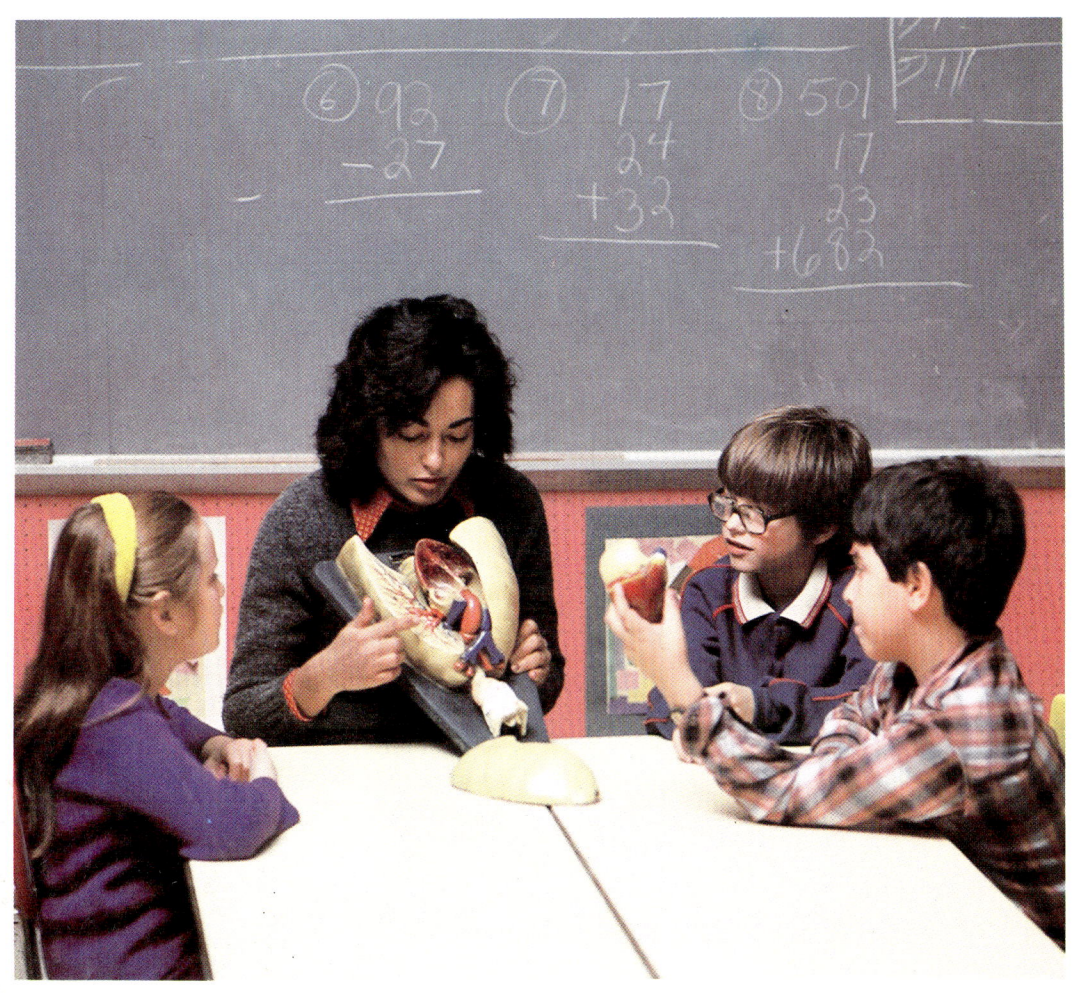

Look at the children on page 26.
How old do you think each child is?
Tell why you think so.

Look at the picture on this page.
In what ways are the children growing?
Why is learning important?

Growing Isn't Just Getting Bigger

Seeing is one of your senses. So is hearing. Touch, smell, and taste are also senses.

Use your senses to help you grow. Watch. Listen. Be willing to taste new foods. Learn about new smells. There is a whole world out there for you. Learn about it and grow.

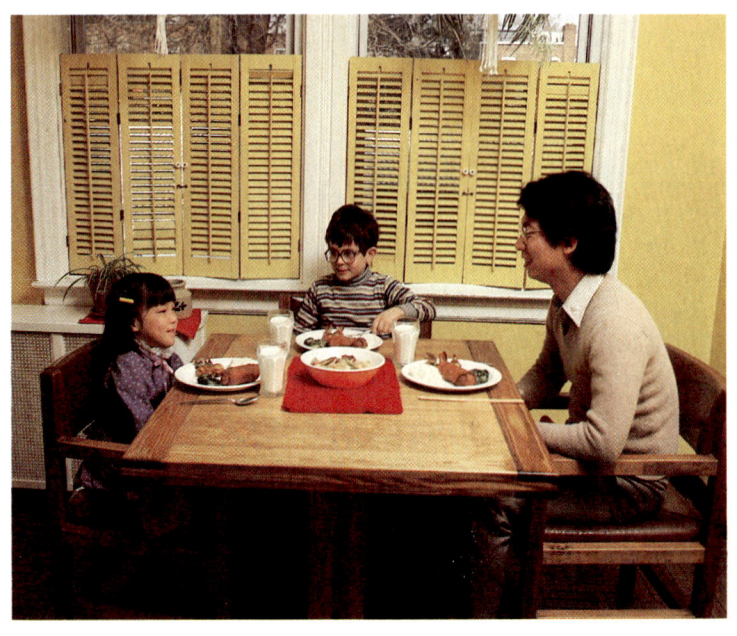
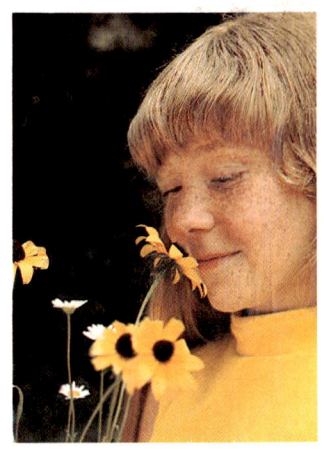

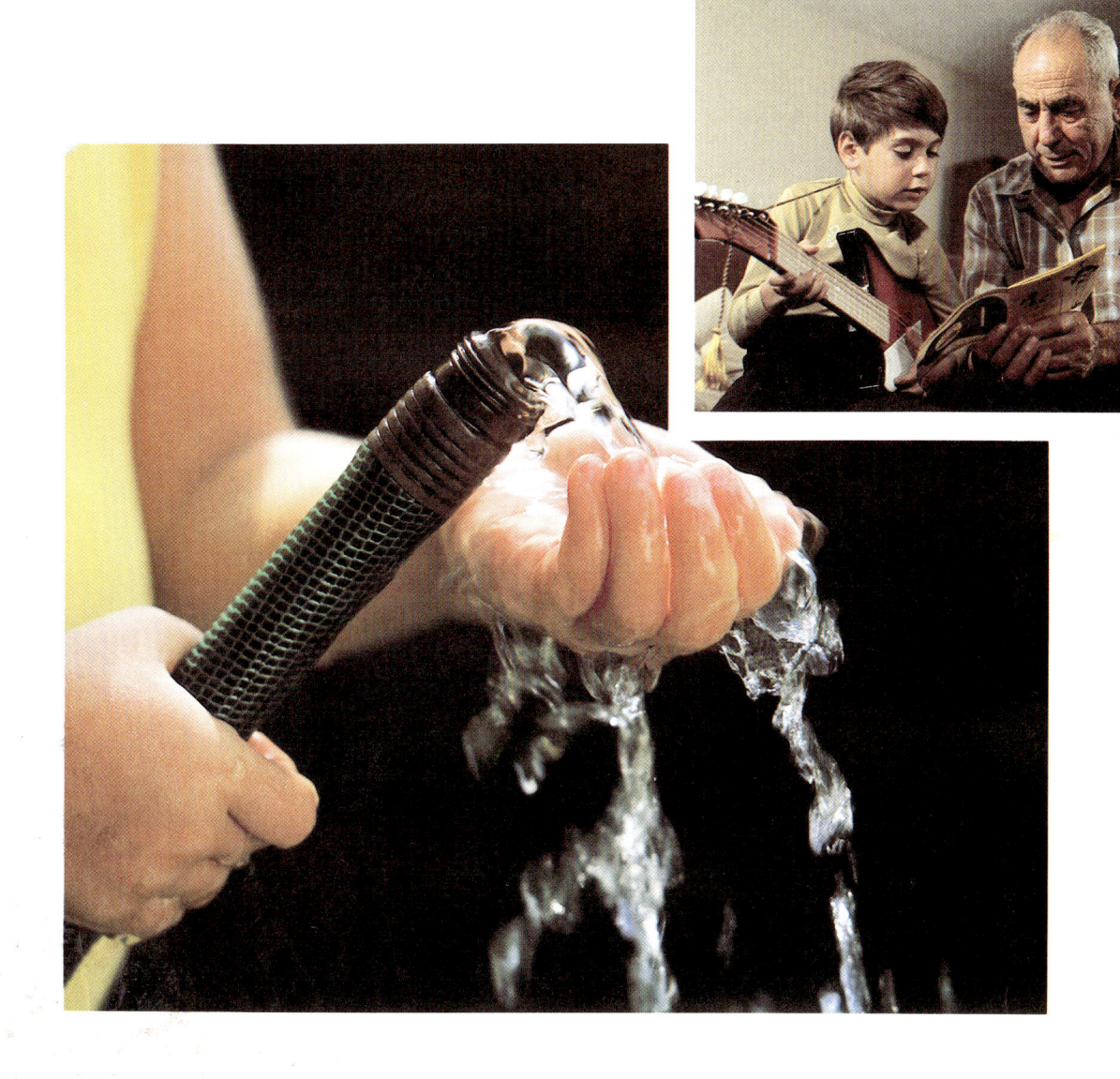

Look at all four pictures.

Which senses are the children using?

How are they using their senses to grow?

Tell other ways to use your senses to grow.

29

Your Eyes and Ears Help You Grow

Use your senses for safety. Use your eyes. Watch where you are going.

Use your ears, too. Listen for sirens. Listen for other special sounds. Know what they mean. Know what to do.

Keeping safe helps keep you growing.

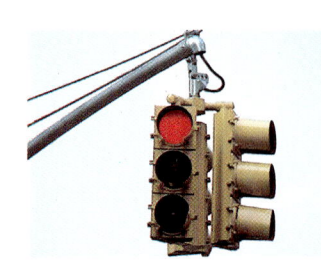

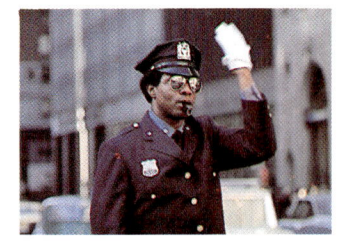

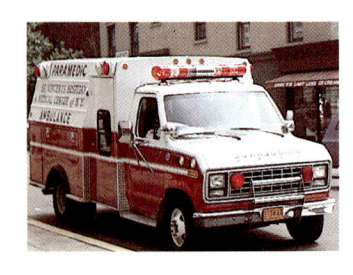

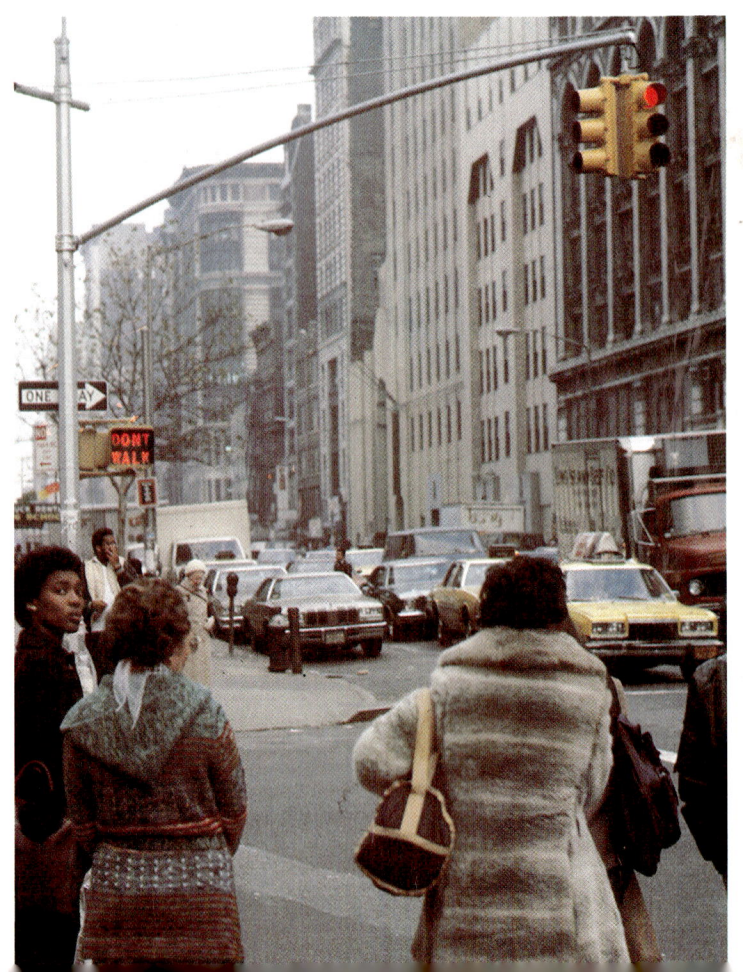

brain

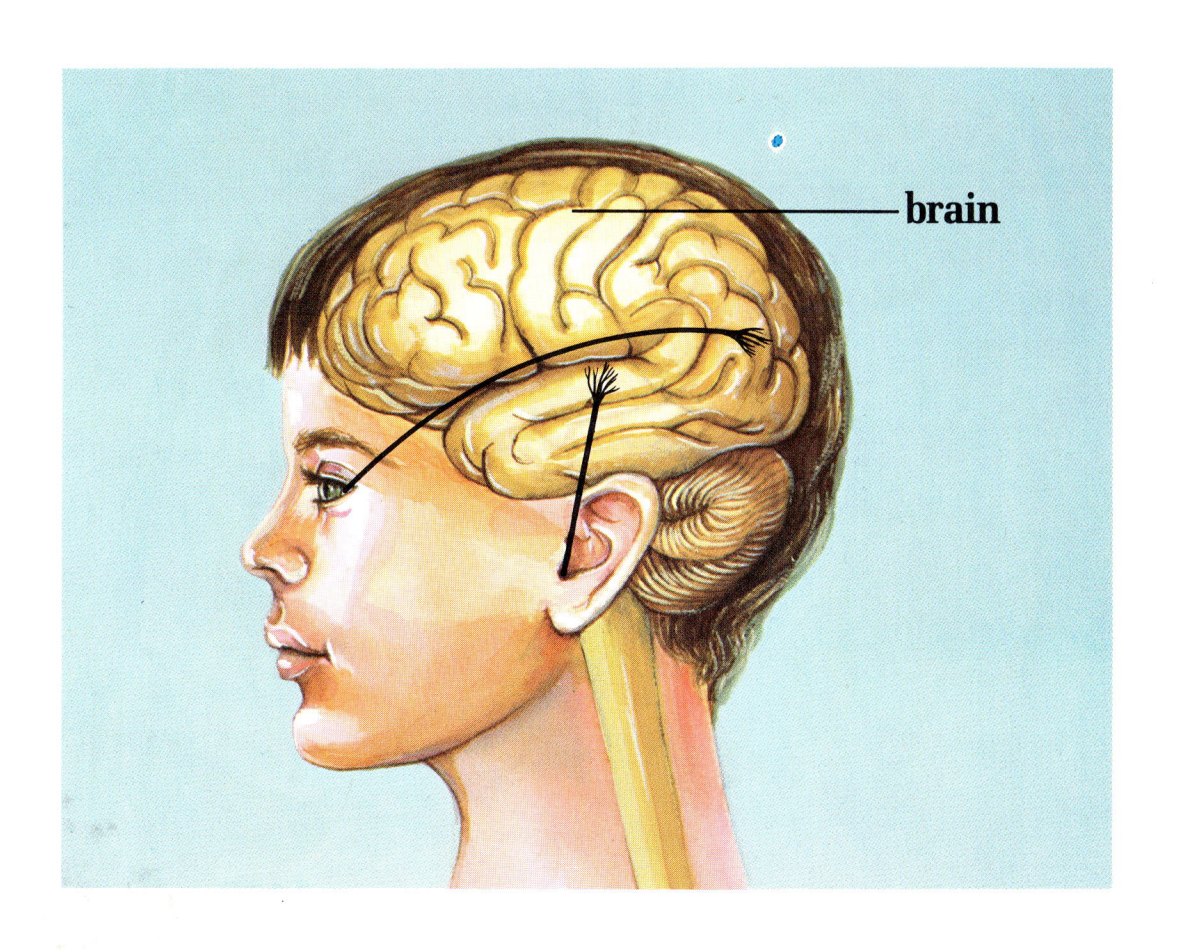

Look at the pictures on page 30.

Which senses can help the people cross the street safely?

How do these senses help?

In what other ways can they help?

Look at the picture on this page.

Which part of the body helps you use your eyes and ears?

Health Highlight

Seeing Colors Differently

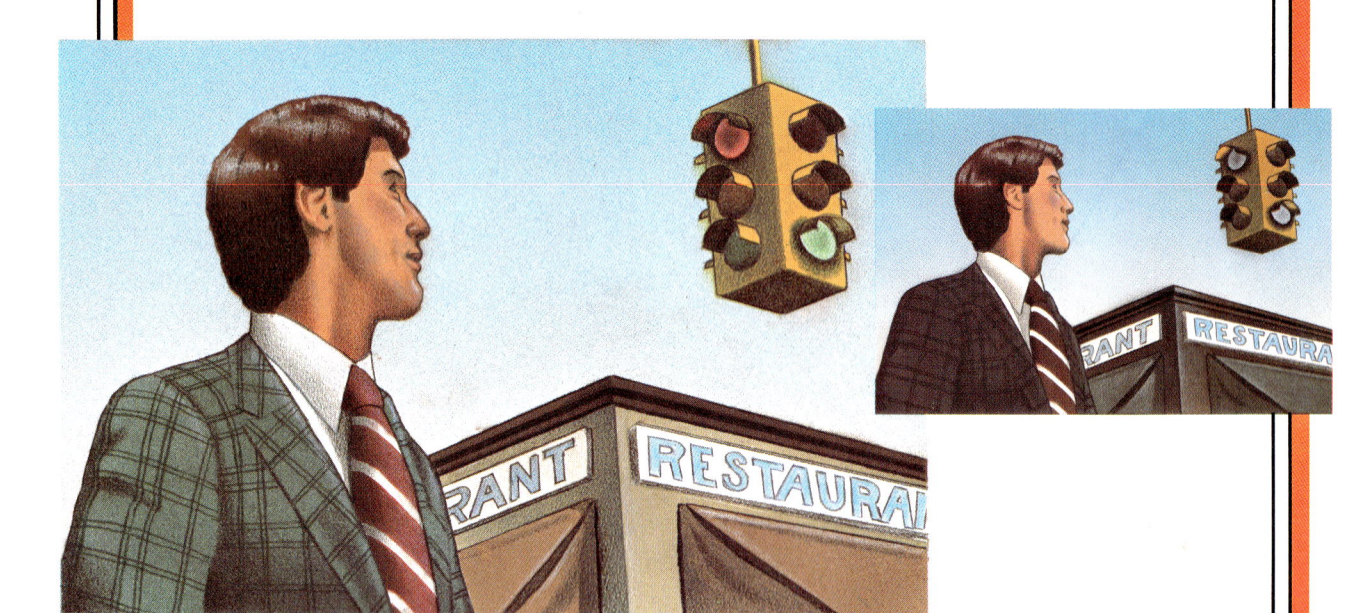

Some people are color-blind. They don't see all colors. Many color-blind people do not see the difference between green and red. Being color-blind does not stop people from seeing well. They just see colors differently.

When are colors important for safety?

Going, Seeing, and Doing

1. Trace your right foot. Go to a classmate. Trade tracings. Tell how each foot is different.

2. Stand against a wall. Put tape on it to show how tall you are. Write the date. Do this every month for five months. See how you have grown.

3. Put a toy in a bag. Trade bags with a friend. Close your eyes. Reach into the bag. Guess what is there. What sense are you using?

Other Senses Help You Grow

Your senses of smell and touch can help keep you safe. Smoke may mean danger. Learn other smells that may mean danger. Know what to do when you smell them. Watch out for things that are too hot or too cold.

Use your senses to help keep you safe. Keeping safe helps you grow.

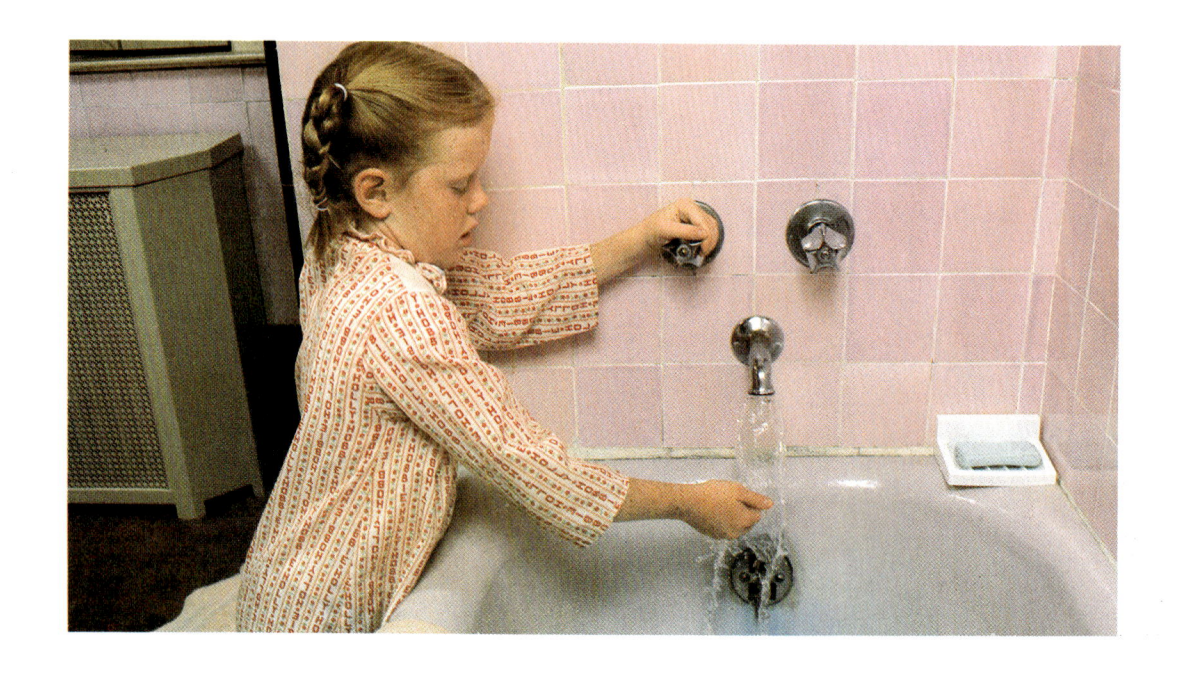

brain

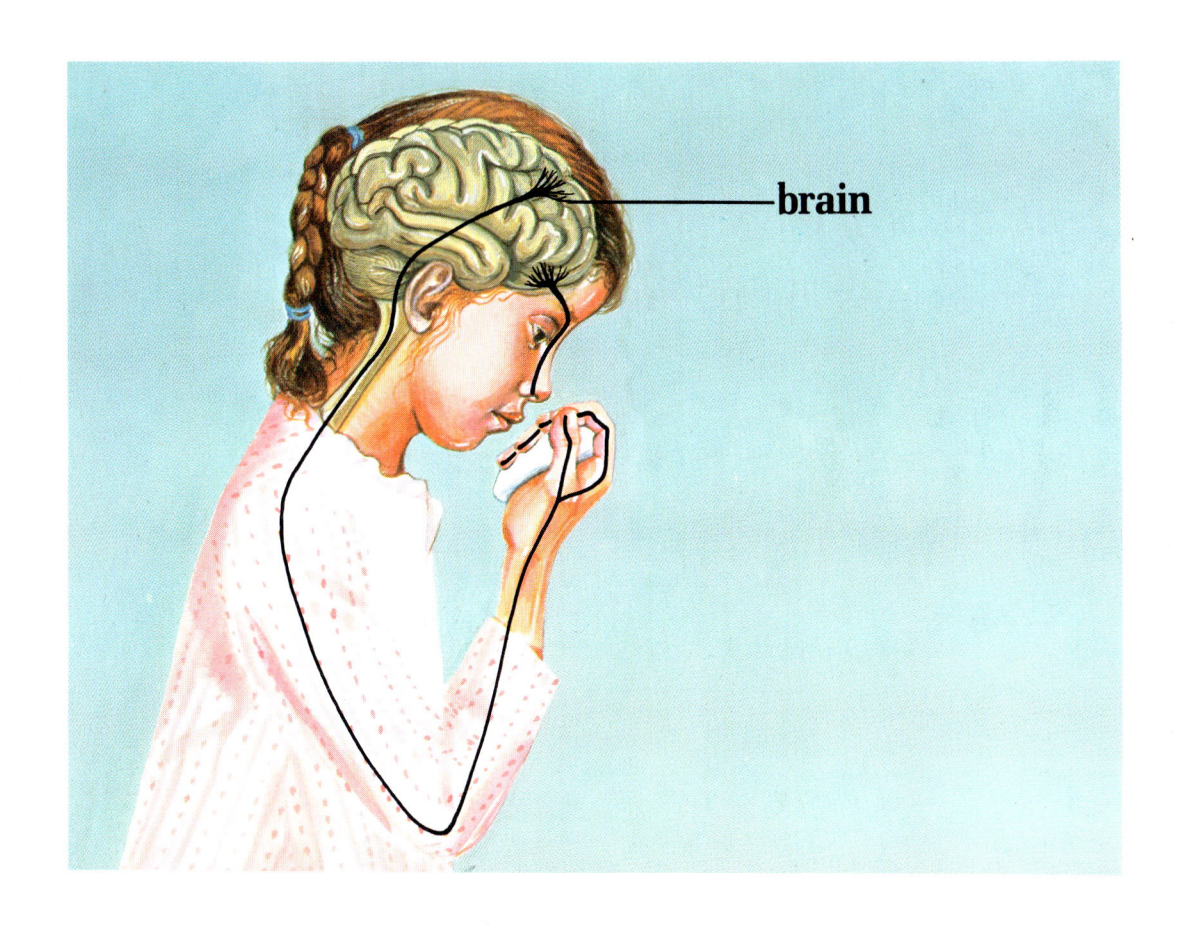

Look at the picture on page 34.

How is the girl using her sense of touch?

Tell how the senses of smell and touch can help with growing.

Look at the picture on this page.

What parts of the body help you use your senses of smell and touch?

35

Health Habits for Growing

It takes energy to grow. Some good health habits help you have the energy you need.

Get exercise every day. Eat healthful meals. Get enough rest and sleep every day.

You are growing all the time. Help your body have energy for growing.

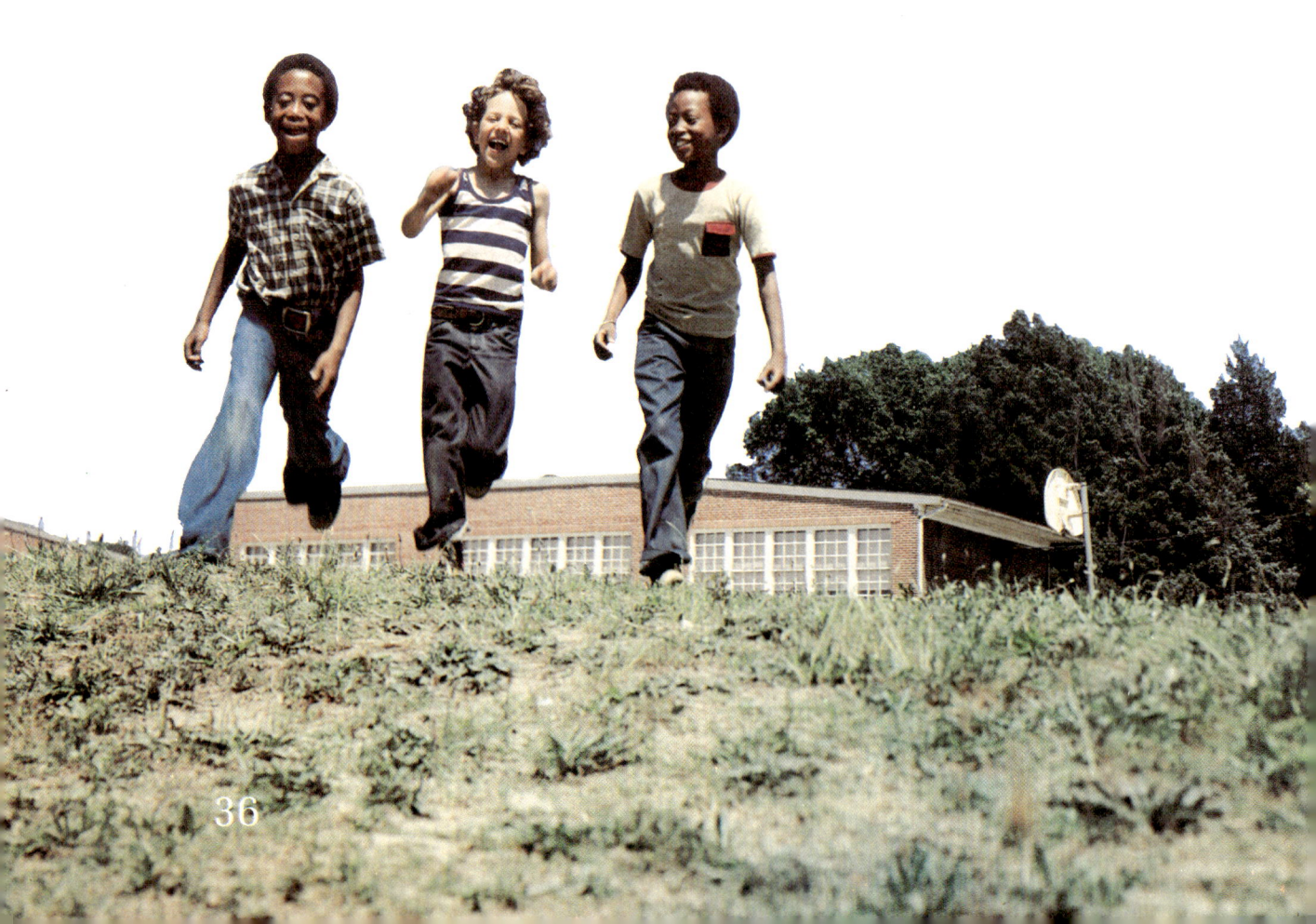

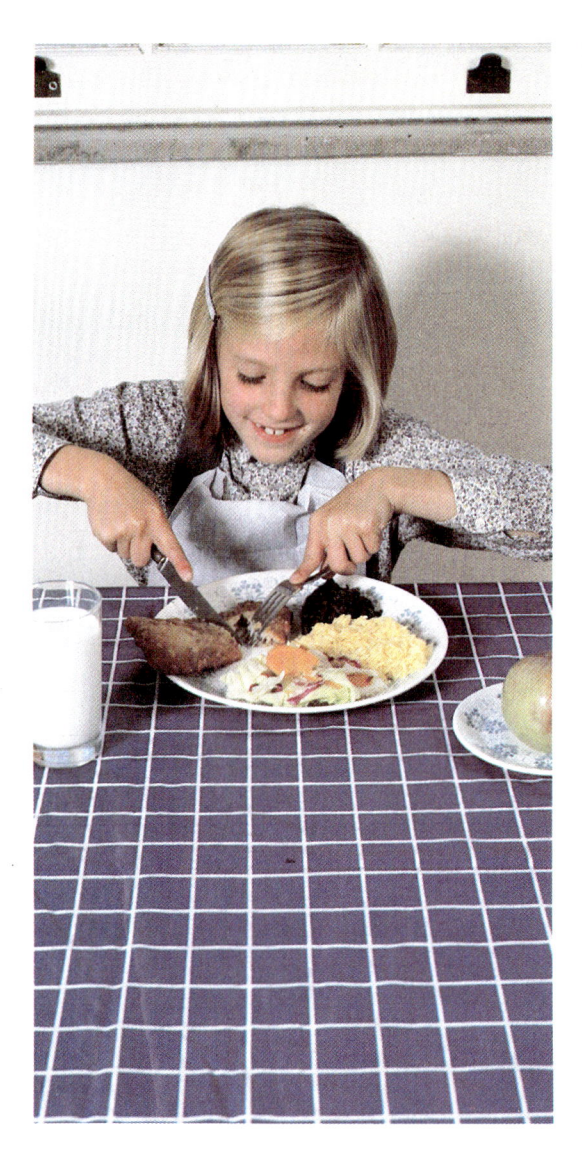

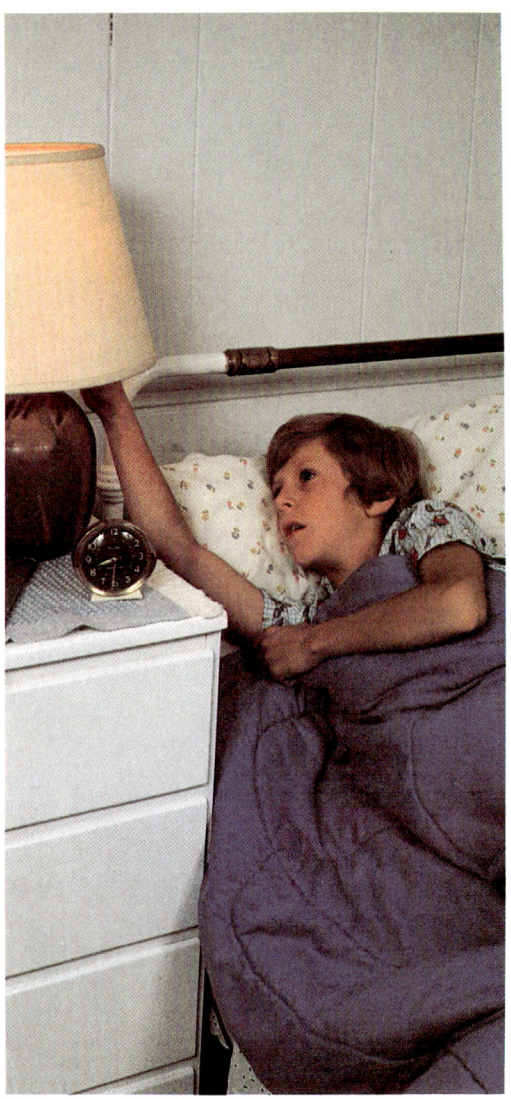

Look at all three pictures.
What are the children doing?
Tell why these are good health habits.
Tell how they help the children grow.
Show ways you can help yourself grow.

More Habits for Growing

Keeping clean helps keep you healthy. Staying healthy helps keep you growing.

Brush your teeth. Brush after eating. Be sure to brush at bedtime.

Wash your hair. Wash it every few days. Keep it looking nice. Keep your whole body clean. Being clean feels good.

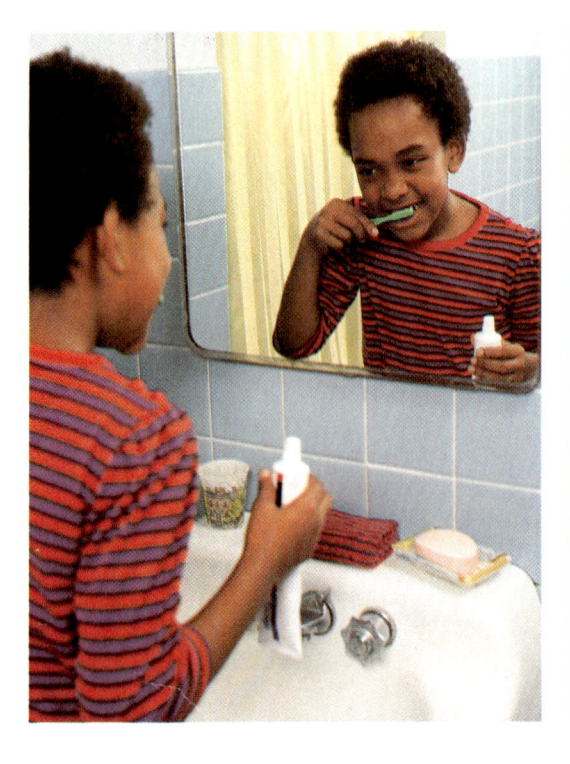

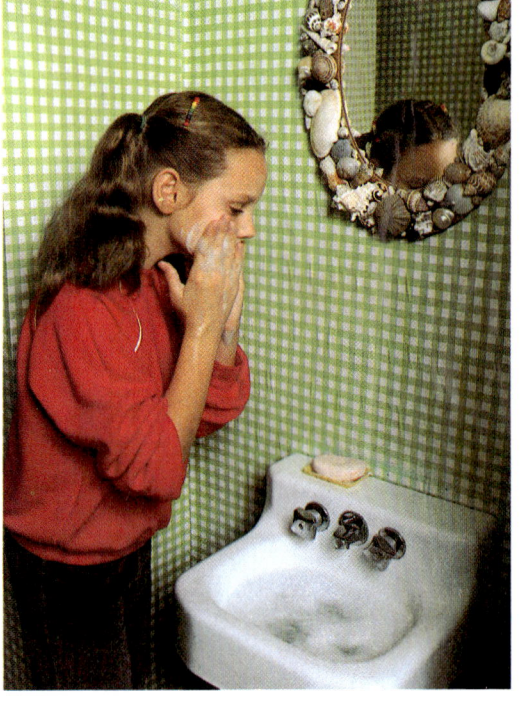

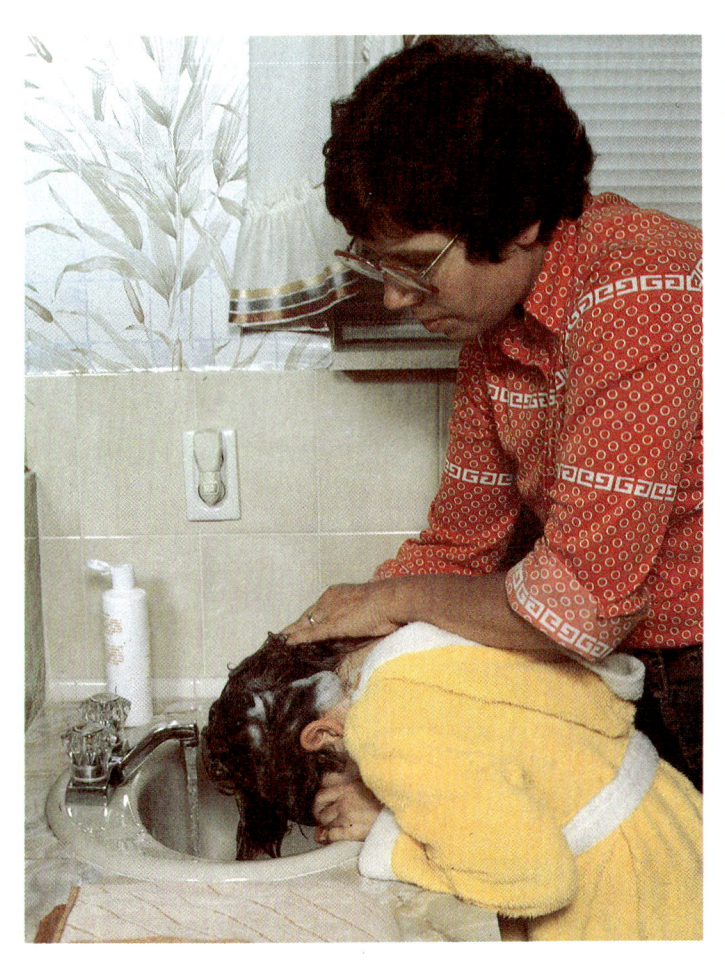

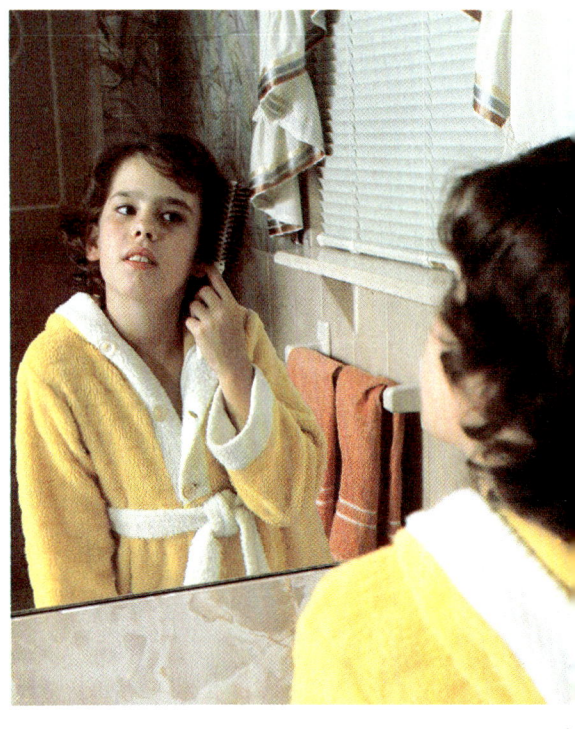

Look at all four pictures.

Name the good health habits.

Tell why these habits are important for growing.

List some other good health habits.

Why are these habits important for growing?

39

Your Turn

Learning and Growing

Jack and his family are visiting Mexico. Jack has never been there before. Many things there are new to him. There is so much to learn.

Help Jack learn and grow.

What kinds of things can he learn about Mexico?

How can his senses help him?

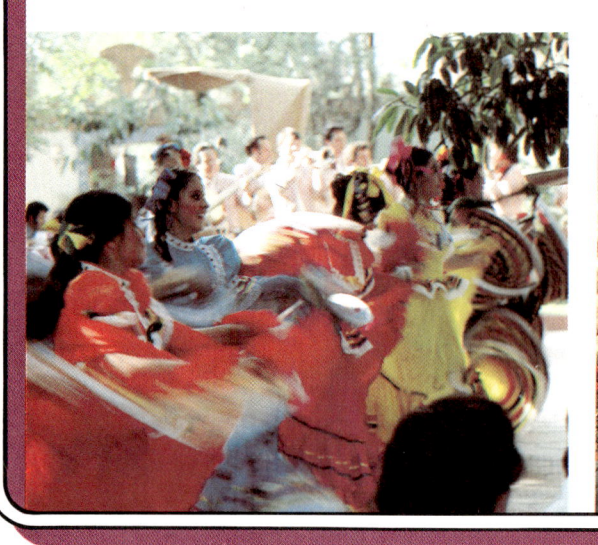

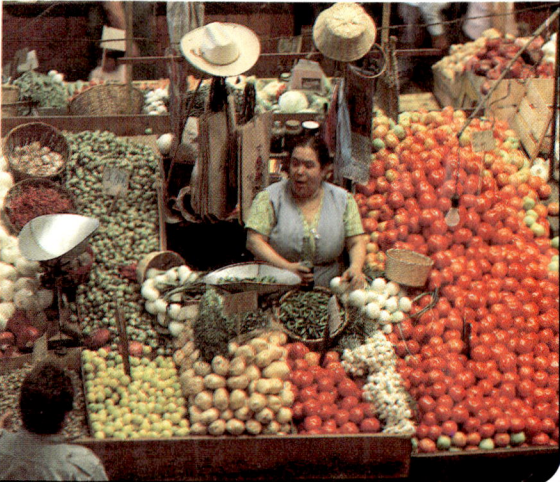

Health in Action

1. Look at the picture. Name the parts of the body.

2. Find pictures of good health habits. Put them into a notebook. Follow their example.

3. Close your eyes. Your teacher will hold something under your nose. Breathe deeply. What do you smell?

4. Think of a place you have visited. Write what you saw and did there. Write about the sounds and smells. Then, trade papers with a friend. Learn about a different place.

Do You Remember?

Your Health Words

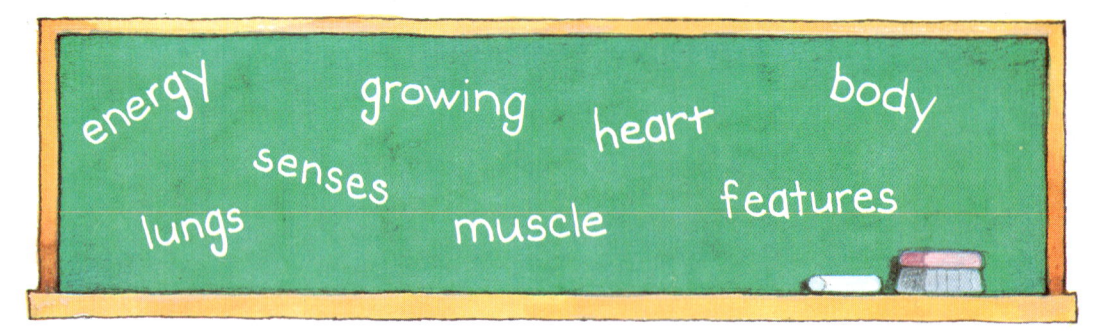

energy growing heart body
senses
lungs muscle features

Answer the questions.

Use the Health Words.

1. What parts of the body are inside?
2. Which word tells about how you look?
3. What can help you grow?

Your Health Ideas

1. Name some of your features.
2. Name some parts of the body that grow.
3. Tell how your senses help you grow.
4. Tell some good health habits for growing.

Health Check-Up

Tell which sentences are true.

1. Everyone is the same.
2. Learning is not a way of growing.
3. Listening can help you grow.
4. You grow only by getting bigger.
5. Your sense of smell can tell you about danger.
6. Reading is the only way to learn.
7. Eating right can help you grow.
8. Sleep cannot help you grow.
9. Washing your hair is a good health habit.
10. Being healthy helps you grow.

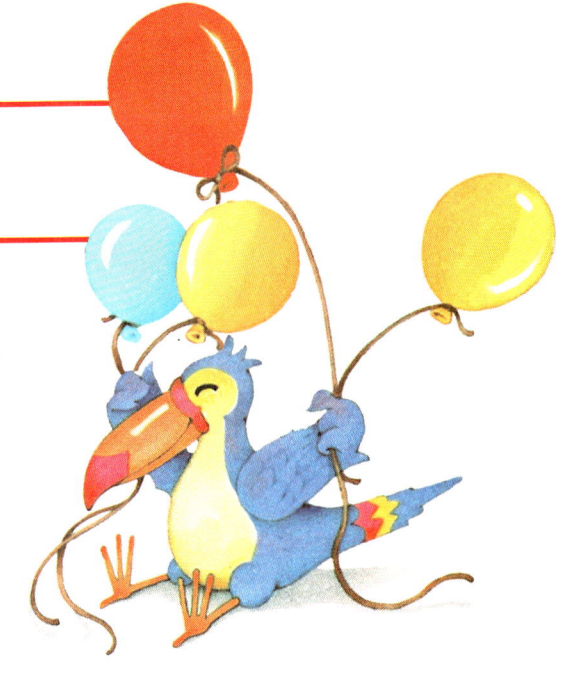

CHAPTER 3

Choosing Your Foods

Different foods help your body in different ways. They help you stay well. Some help your body grow. Others give you energy. You need these different foods. Eat them every day. Help yourself stay healthy.

What are some foods for good health?

Health Words

food groups   milk
fruit   cereal
vegetable   grains
meat   diet

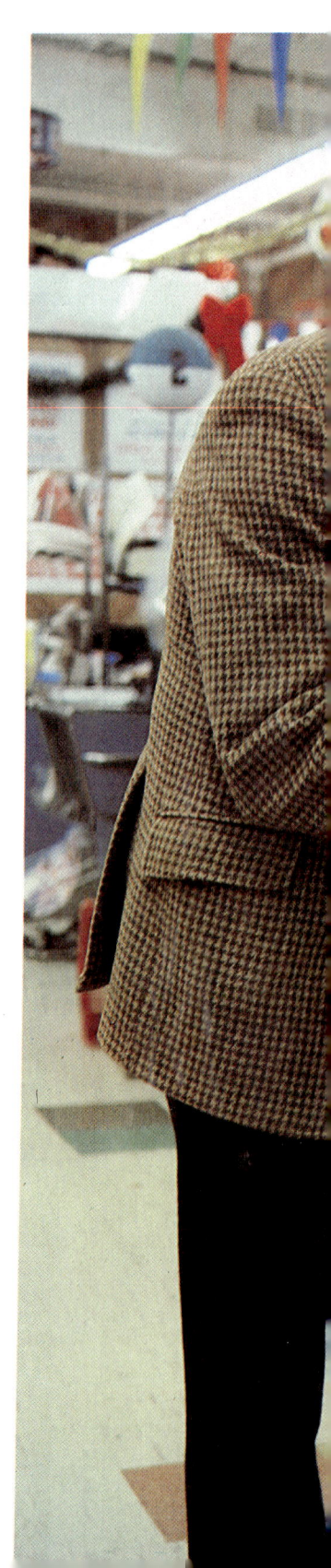

45

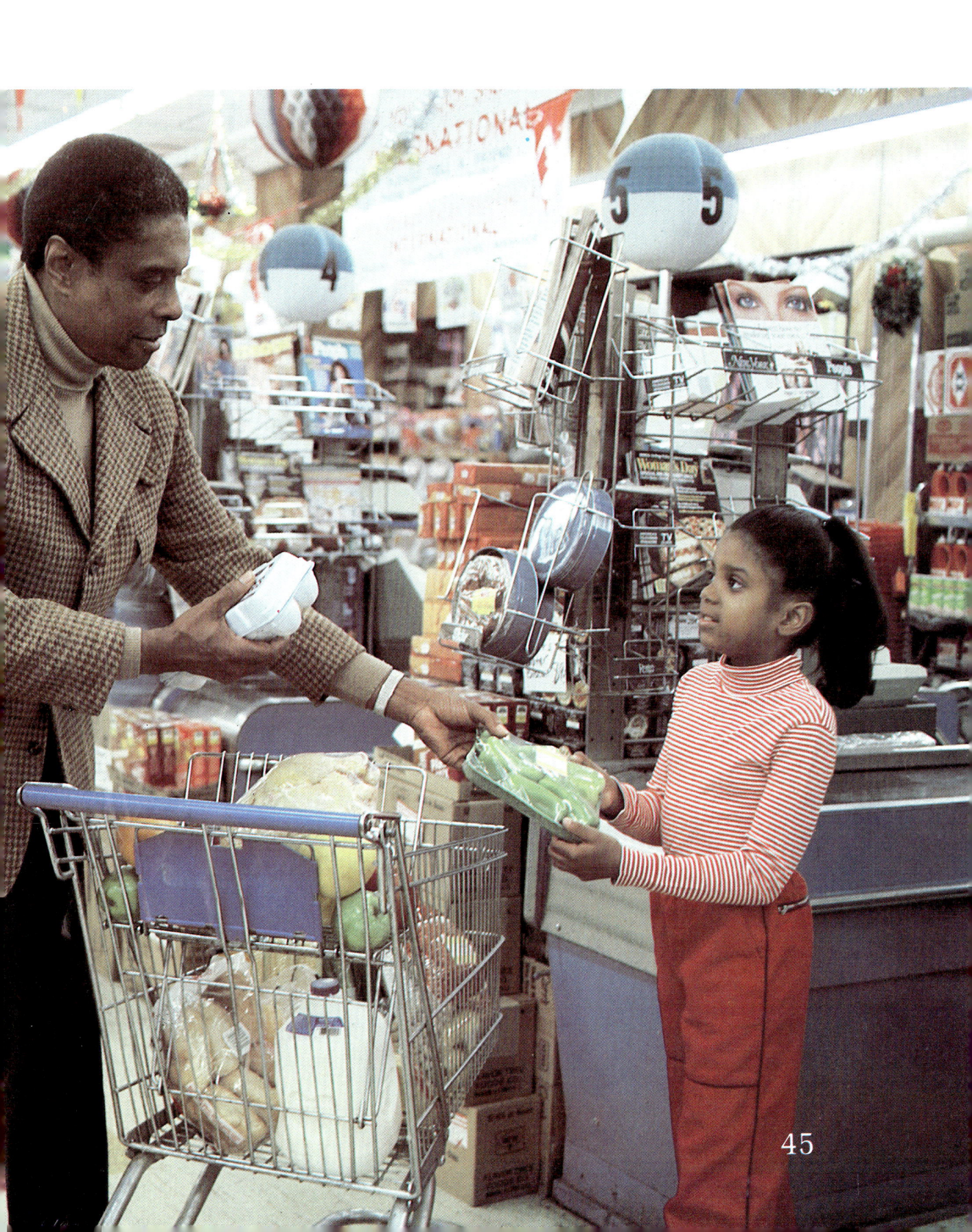

Different Foods

There are four food groups. The fruit and vegetable group is one. The meat group is another. The milk group is a third. The bread and cereal group is a fourth.

You need foods from each food group every day. Your family can help you decide which foods are best for you.

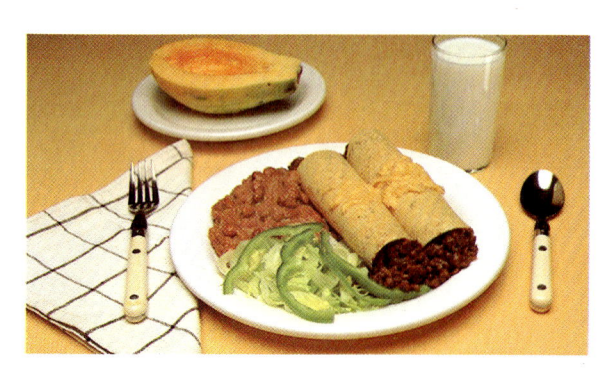

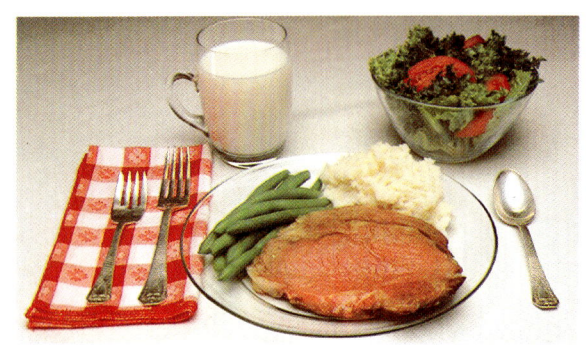

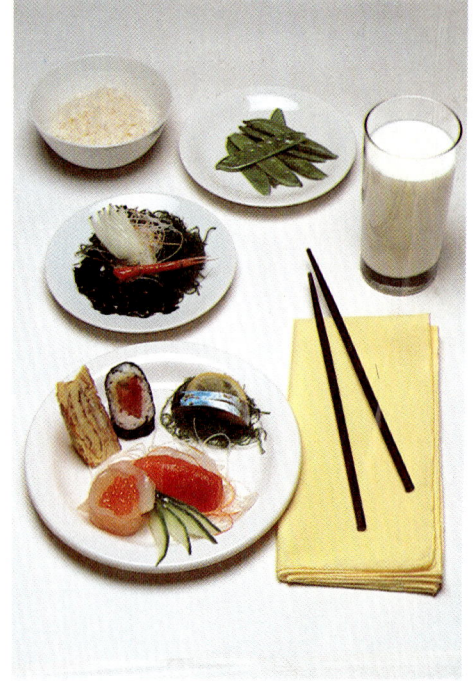

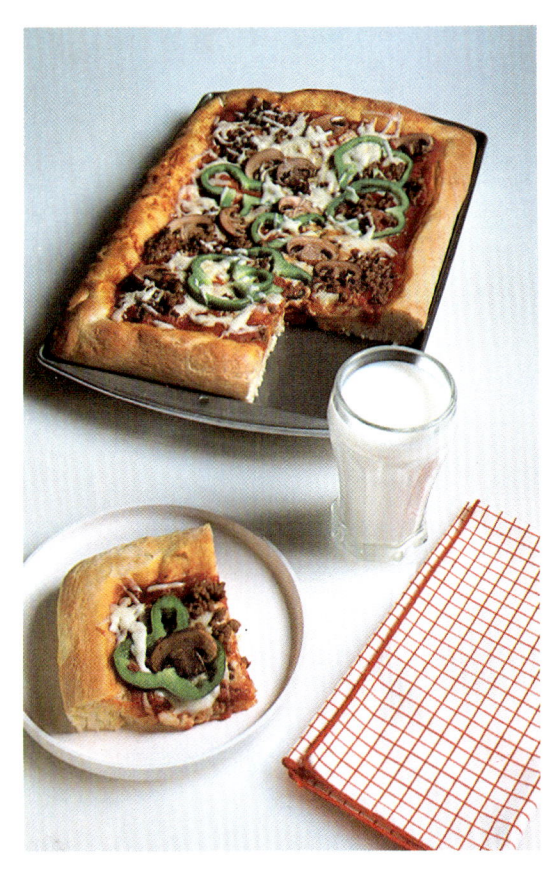

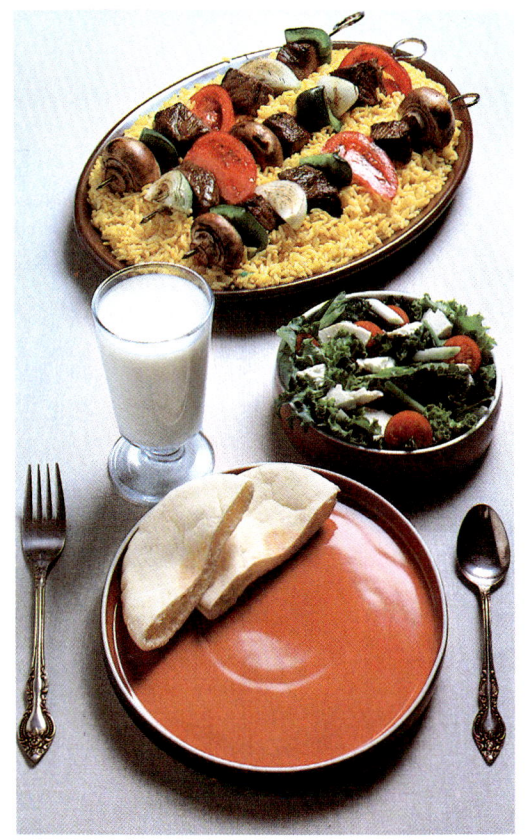

Look at the pictures on both pages.

Name the different kinds of food.

Which of the foods have you eaten?

Which do you like best?

Which would you like to try?

What kinds of food should you eat every day?

Why should you eat these foods?

Foods for Health

The Fruit and Vegetable Group

Eat four or more servings of fruits and vegetables every day. These foods help keep you healthy. They help your eyes and skin. They are good for your teeth and gums, too.

Eat green and yellow vegetables. Eat different kinds of fruit. Eat them every day.

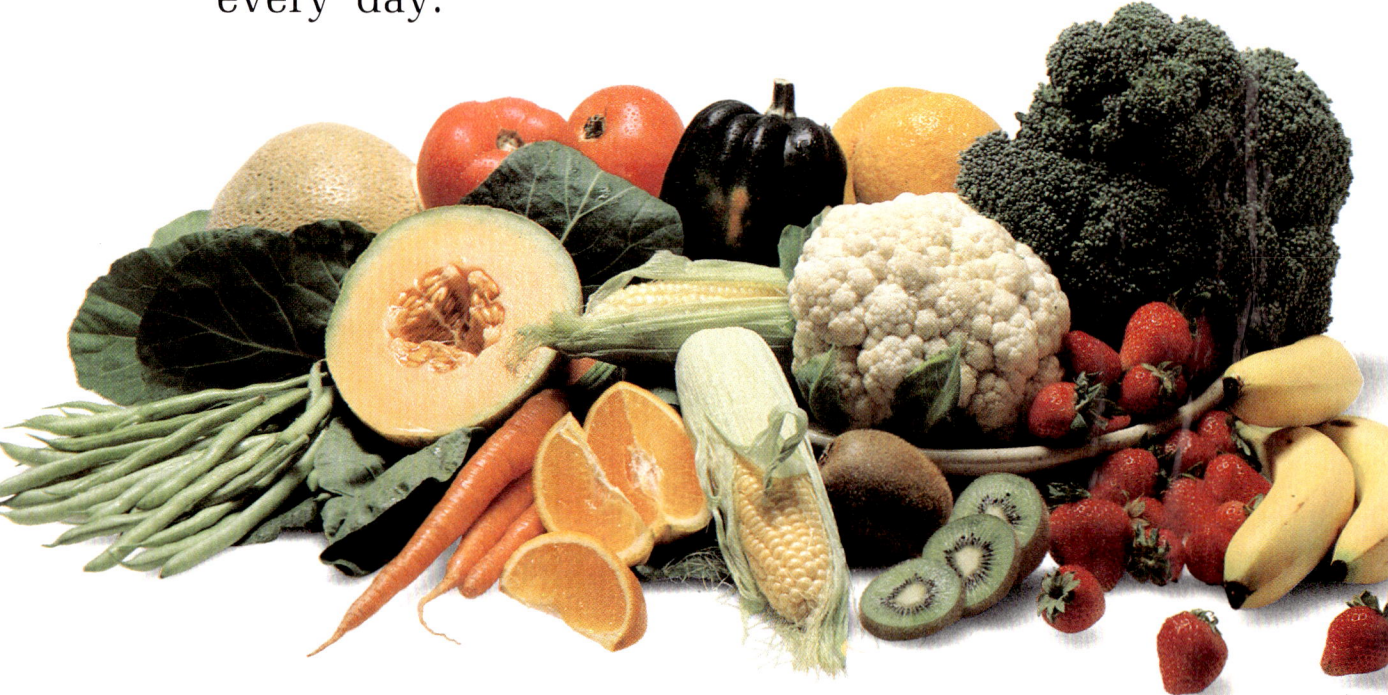

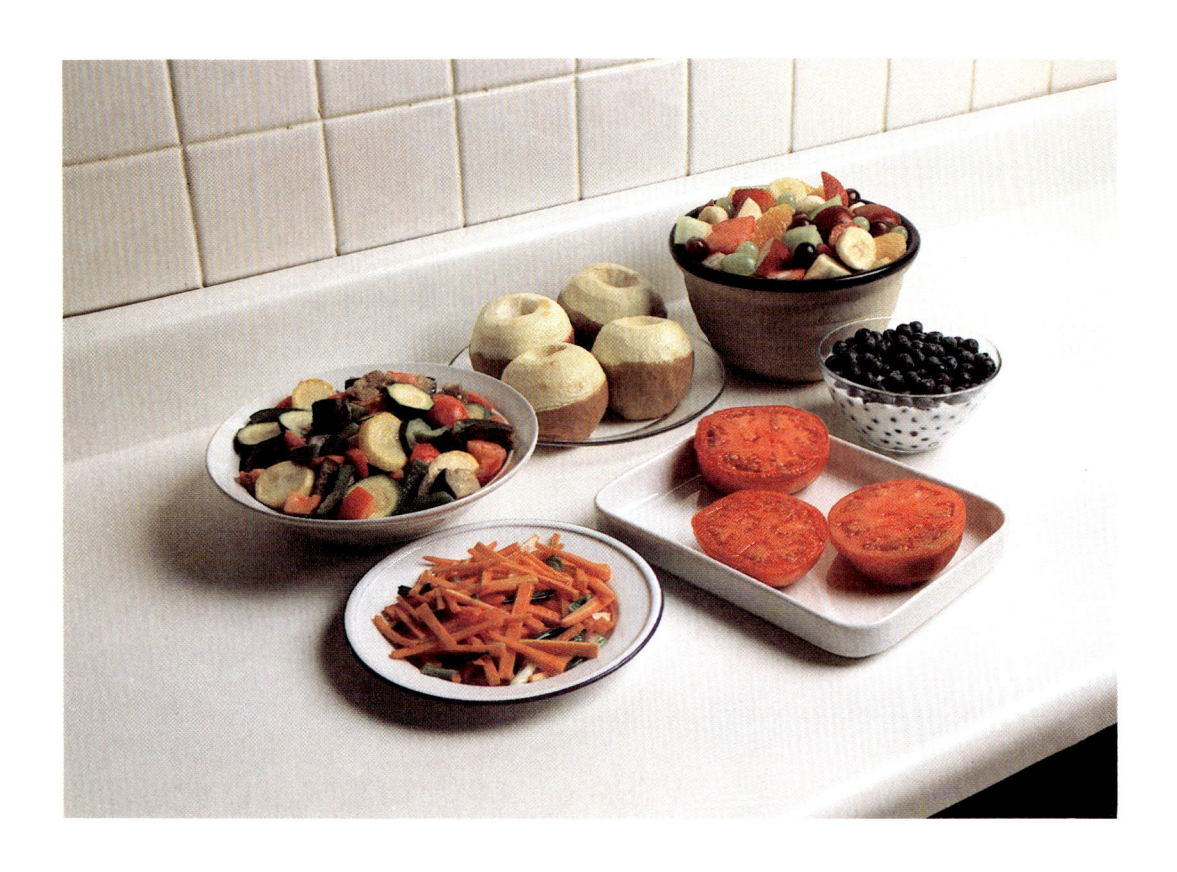

Look at the pictures on both pages.

Name the fruits and vegetables.

Tell which you have eaten.

Tell which you would like to try.

Name other fruits and vegetables.

How many servings of these foods should you eat every day?

Tell why fruits and vegetables are important for good health.

Foods for Health

The Meat Group

There is more to the meat group than just meat. Fish and eggs are in this food group. Chicken and turkey are, too. So are nuts and beans.

All these foods help your body in the same way. They help you grow. They help build muscles. You need two or more servings every day.

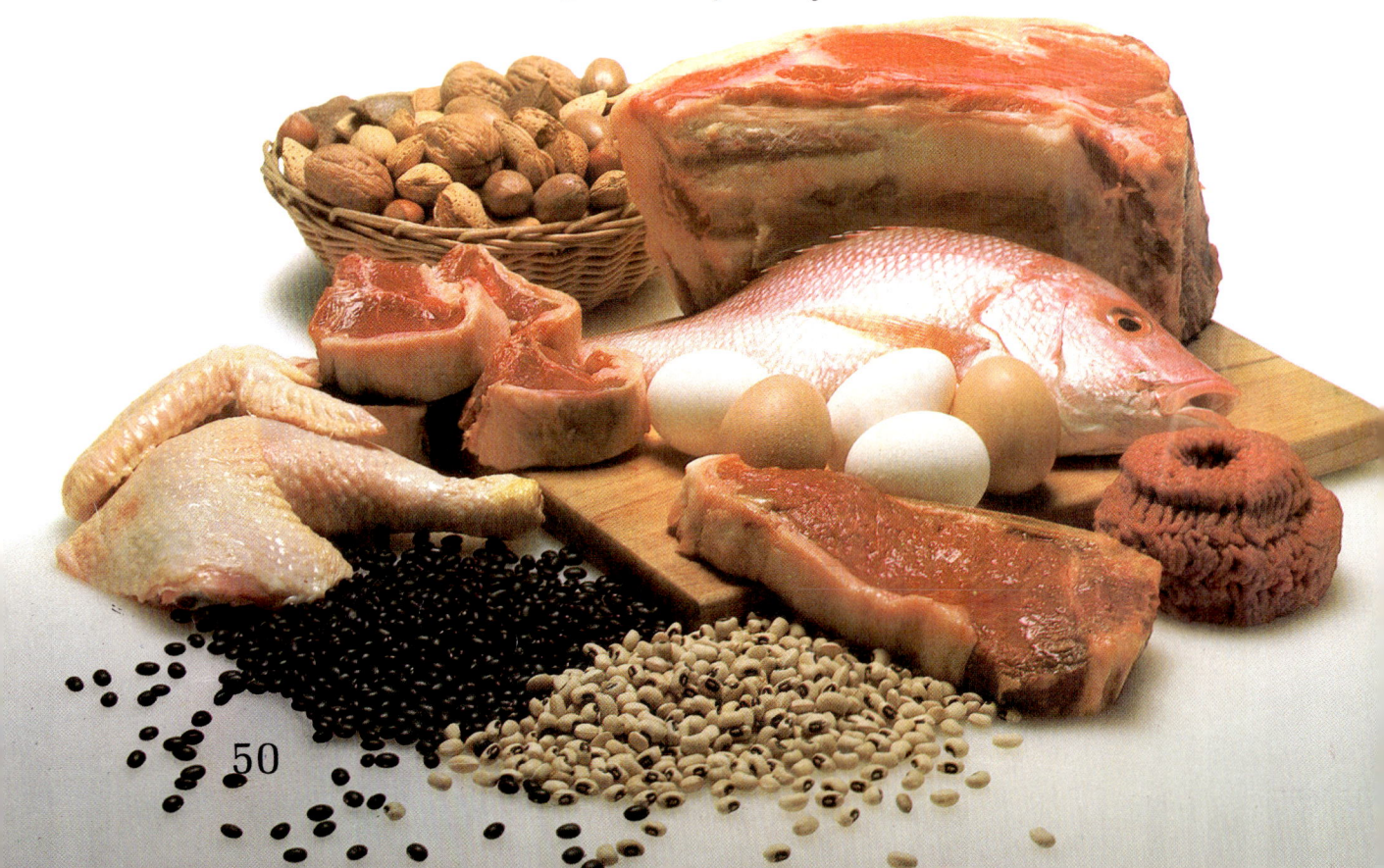

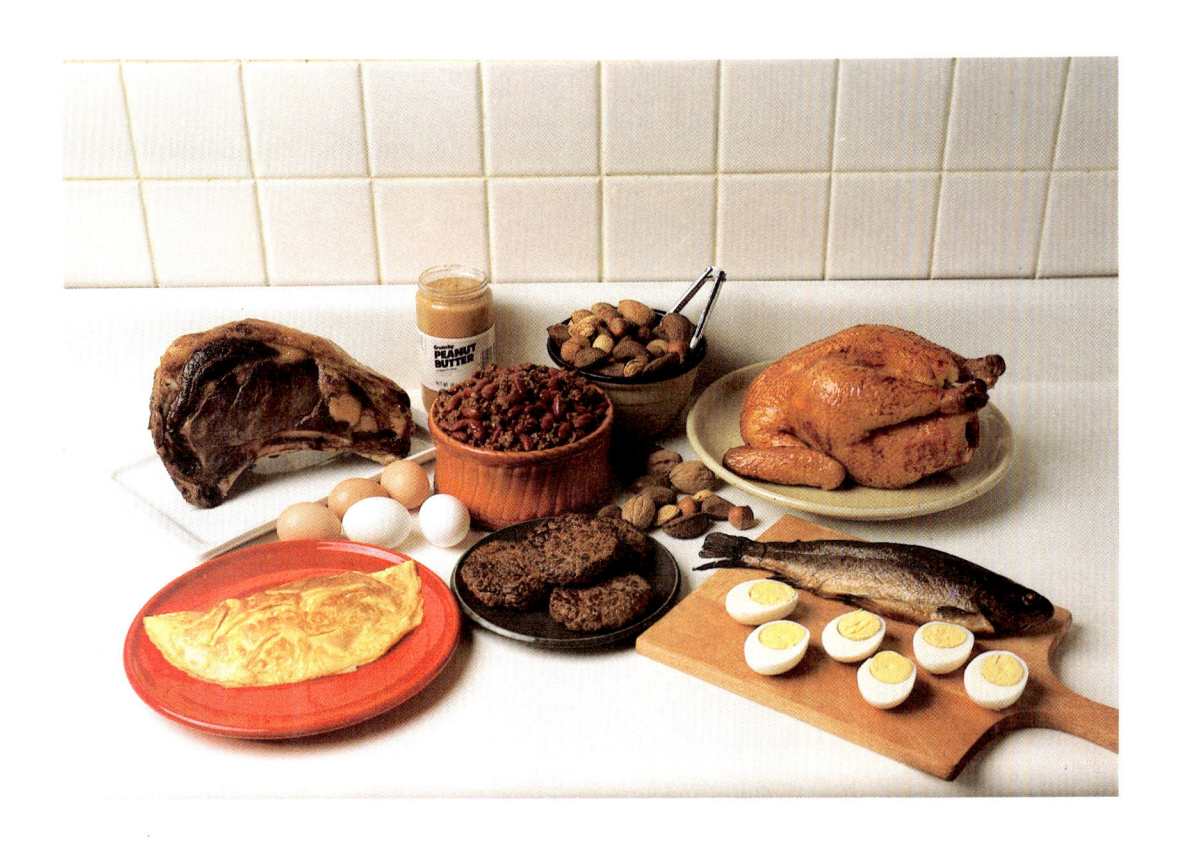

Look at the picture on page 50.
Name the foods.

Look at the foods on this page.
Which have you eaten?
Name other foods in the meat group.
How do foods in the meat group help your body?
How many servings should you eat each day?

Foods for Health

The Milk Group

Foods in the milk group help you grow. They help your teeth and bones stay healthy.

You need two to three cups of milk each day. You can drink milk. You can eat foods made with milk.

Be sure you have enough foods from the milk group every day.

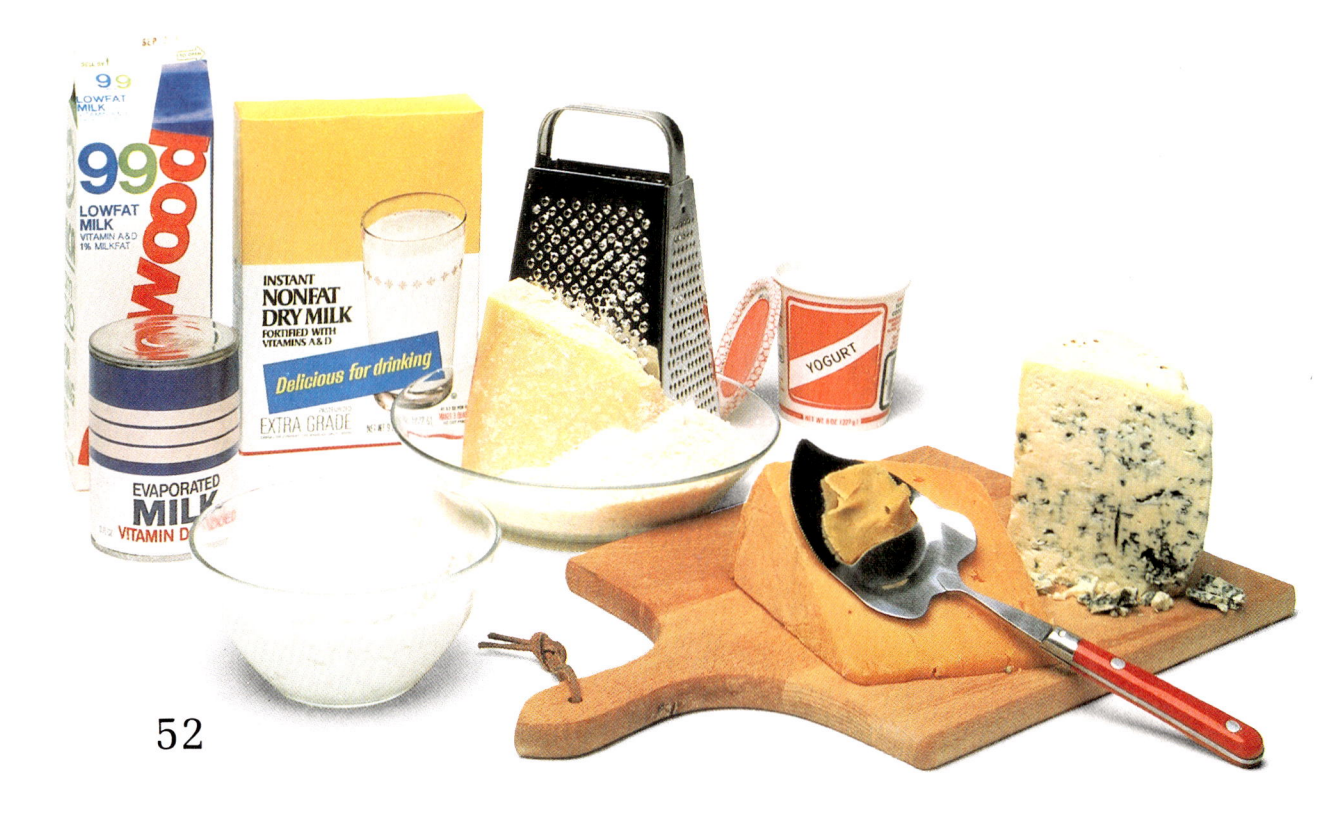

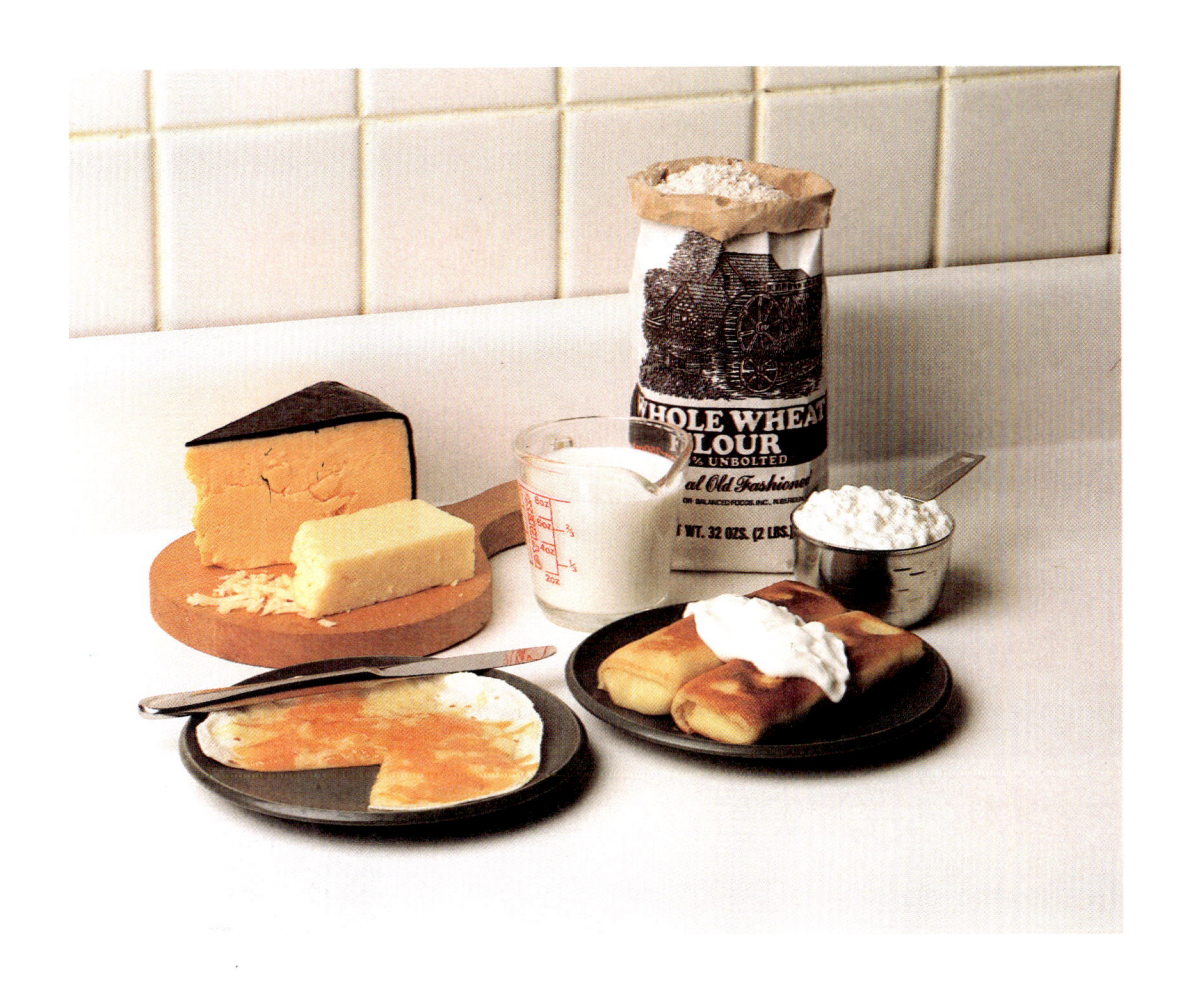

Look at the picture on page 52.

Which of the foods have you tasted?

Look at the dishes of food on this page.

How can you tell they are healthful?

How else can you get the milk you need?

How much do you need every day?

How does milk help your body?

Foods for Health

The Bread and Cereal Group

Foods in the bread and cereal group are made from plants called grains. Wheat and rice are grains. Oats is a grain, too.

Grain foods help give you energy. You need four servings of these foods every day. Choose grain foods you like. Try new ones. Eat grain foods every day.

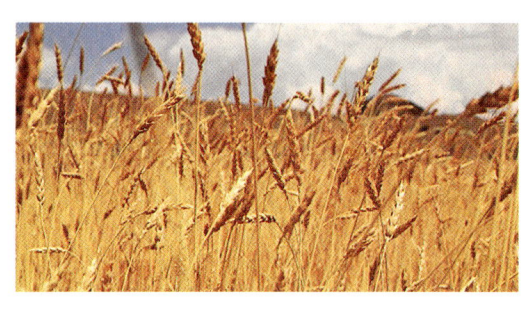

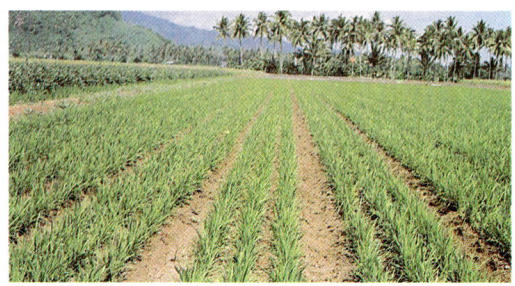

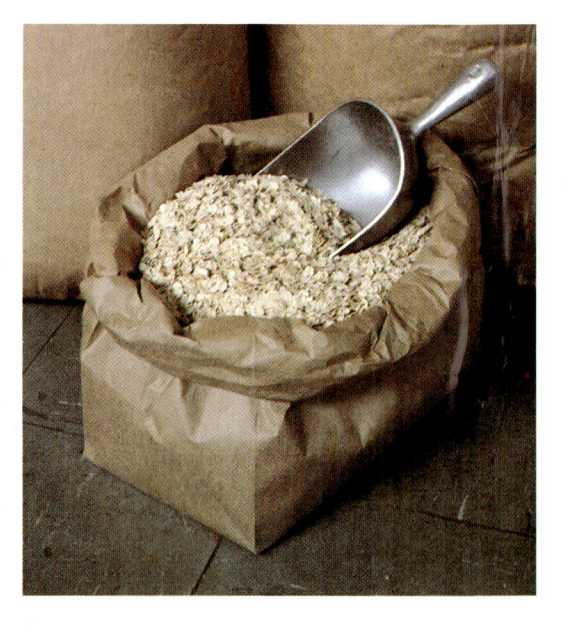

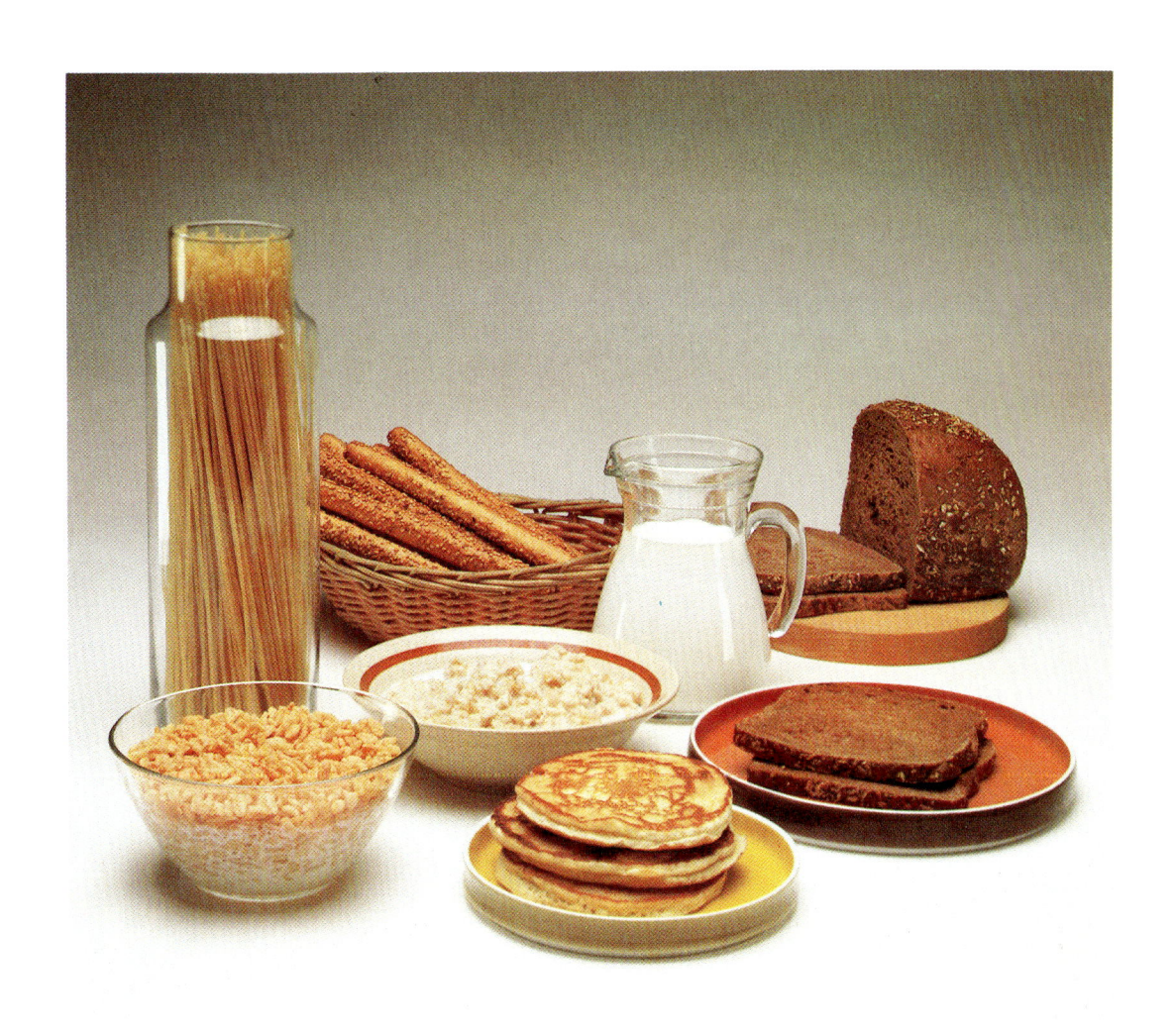

Look at the pictures on page 54.
They show wheat, rice, and oats.

Look at the picture on this page.
Name the foods that come from grains.

How do these foods help your body?

55

Health Highlight

Krill for Lunch

Before long, you may be eating krillburgers instead of hamburgers. Krill are tiny animals. They live in the sea. They look like shrimp. Krill are in the meat group.

Whales eat krill by the ton. Soon you may be eating krill, too. Some people in other countries already are.

How do you think a krillburger would taste?

How can krill help your body?

Going, Seeing, and Doing

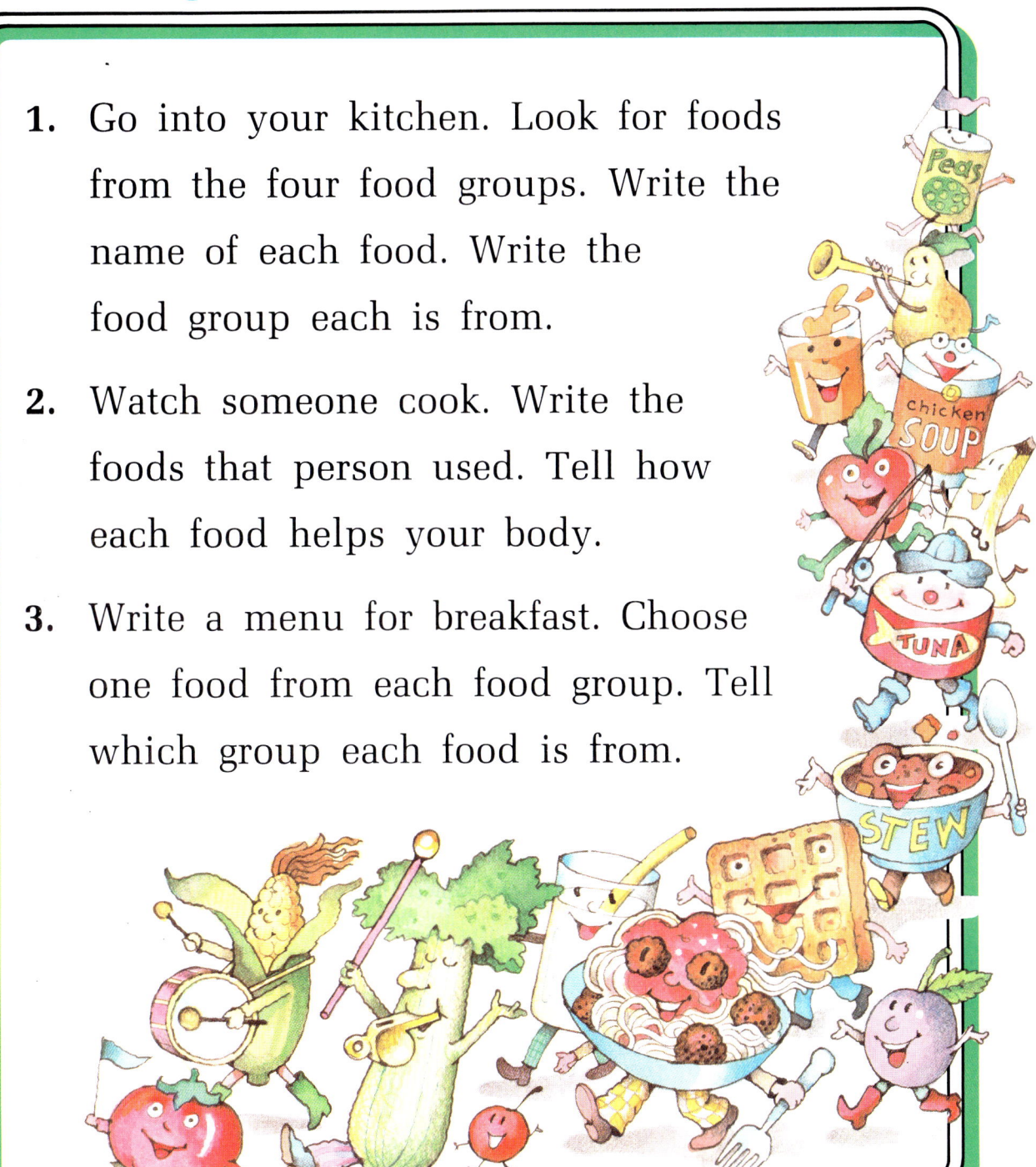

1. Go into your kitchen. Look for foods from the four food groups. Write the name of each food. Write the food group each is from.

2. Watch someone cook. Write the foods that person used. Tell how each food helps your body.

3. Write a menu for breakfast. Choose one food from each food group. Tell which group each food is from.

Healthful Meals

Your diet is what you eat and drink. Be sure your diet is good for you. A good diet helps your body grow. It helps you have energy. It helps you stay healthy.

Drink water. Eat healthful foods at mealtime. Eat different foods. Choose foods from the four food groups.

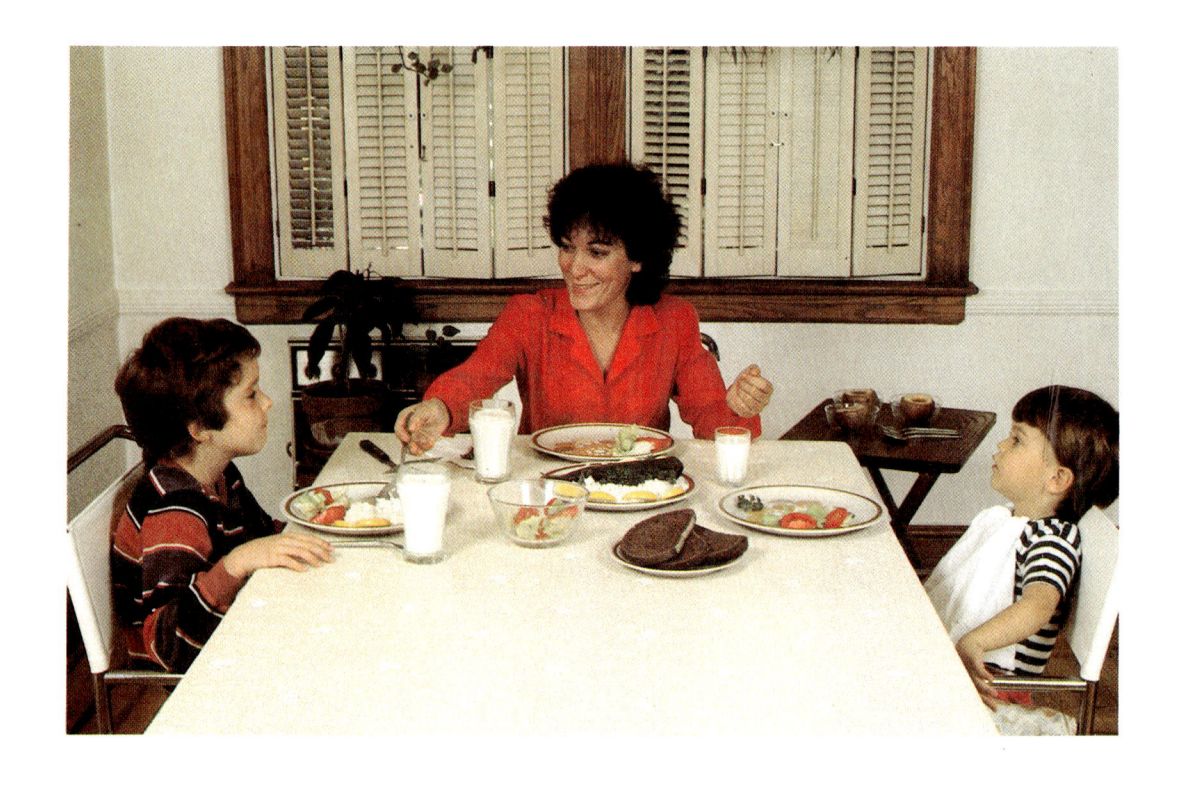

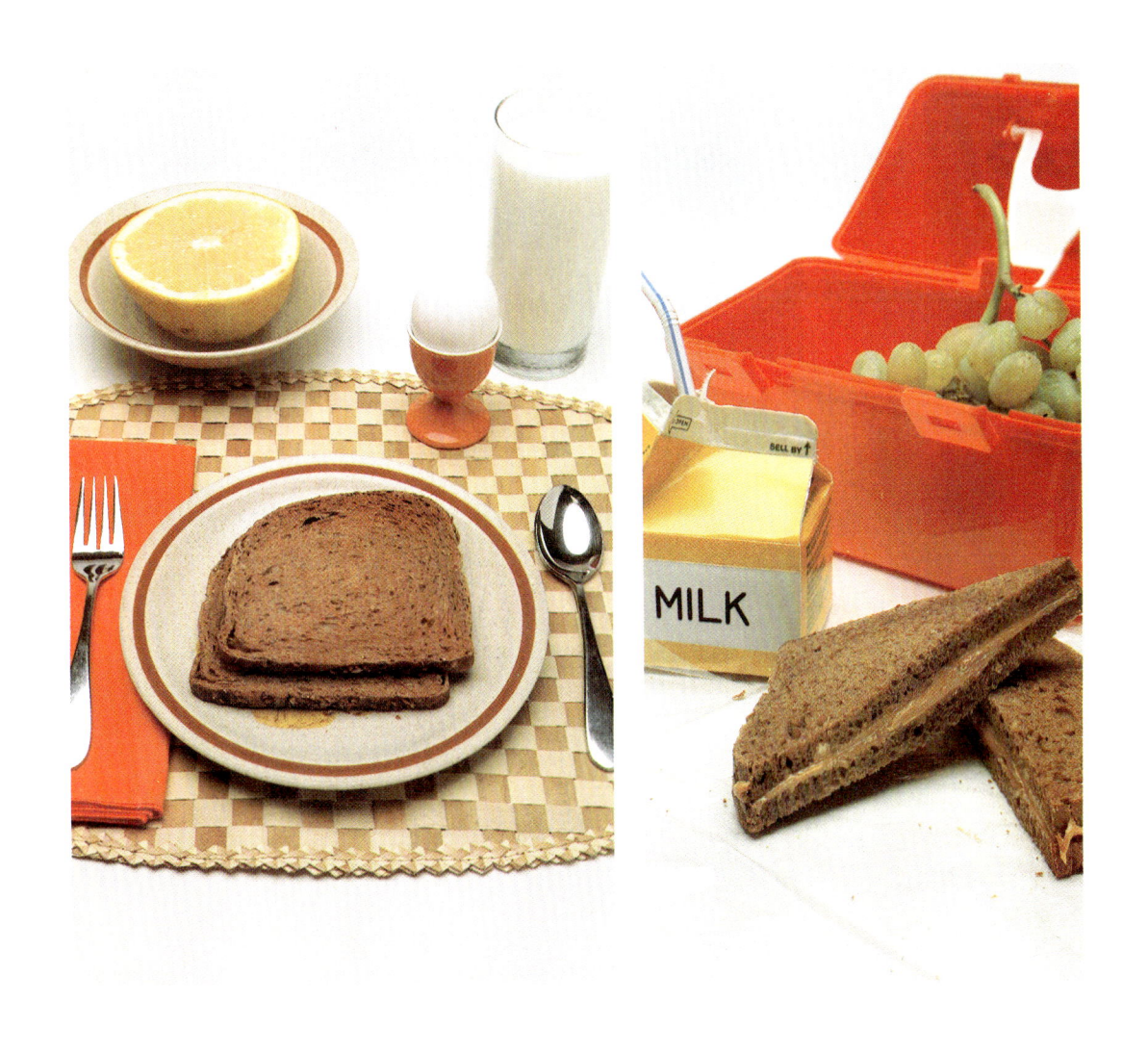

Look at the picture on page 58.
Tell why the meal is healthful.

Look at the two meals on this page.
Tell why each meal is healthful.
Name foods for a healthful meal.
Tell why the meal is healthful.

Snacks and Your Health

Sometimes you might be hungry between meals. You might ask for a snack. Think carefully about what you ask for. Foods from the four food groups make good snacks. These foods help your body stay strong and healthy. They are good for you at mealtimes. They are good for you as snacks.

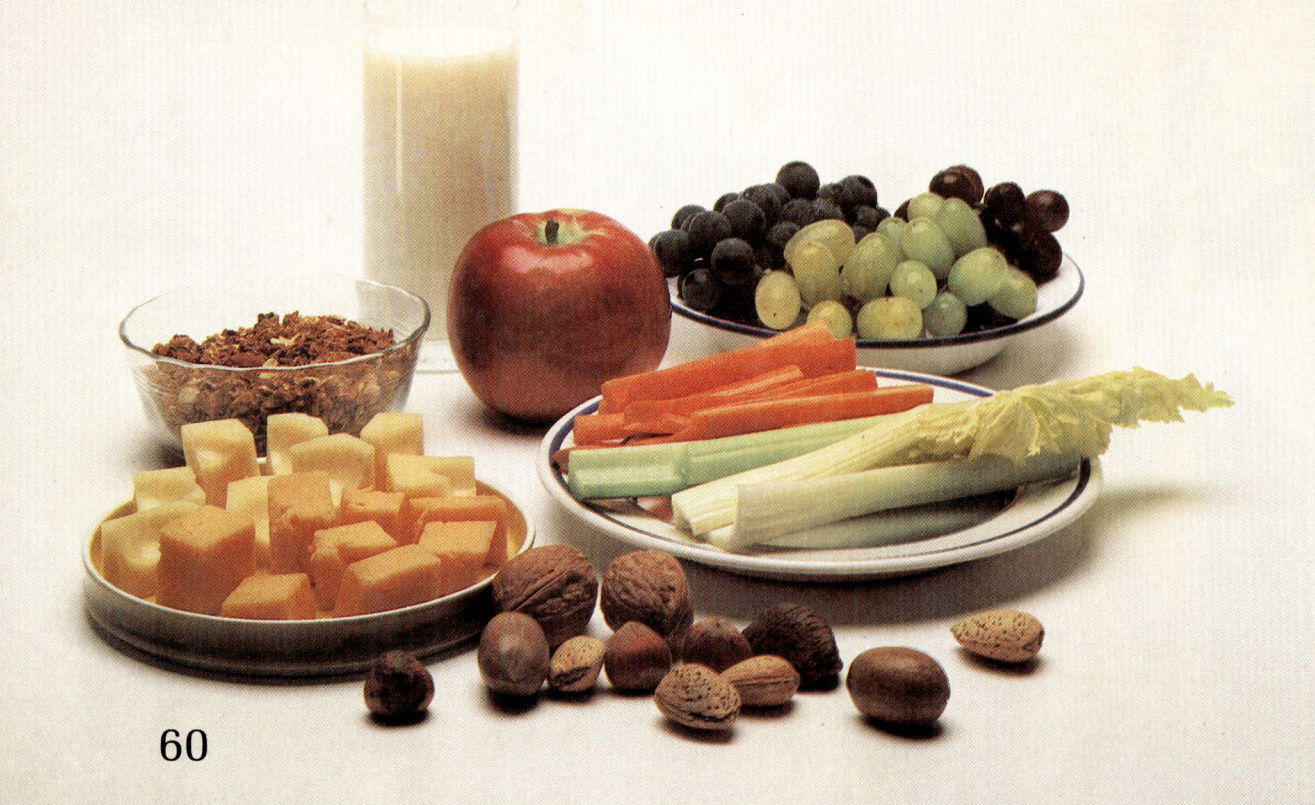

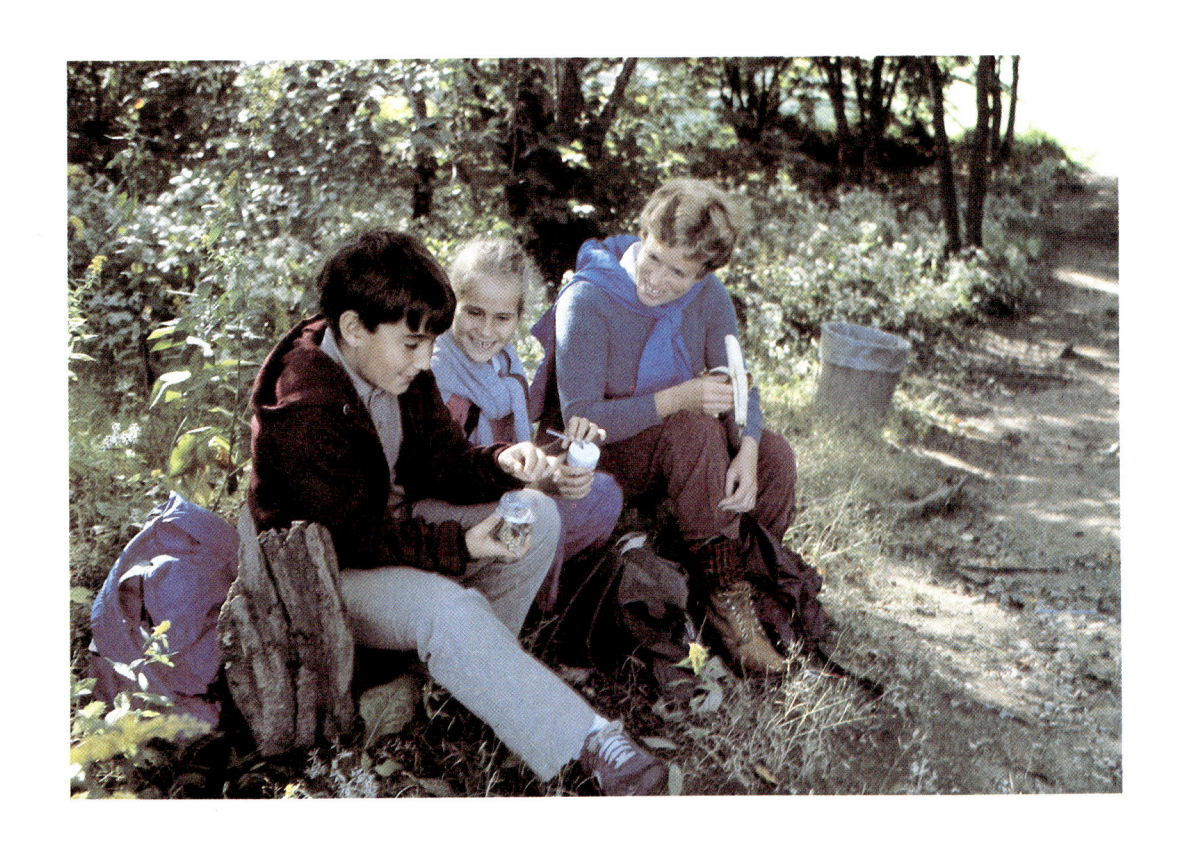

Look at the picture on page 60.

Tell the food group each snack comes from.

Name other healthful snacks.

Look at the picture on this page.

What snack foods do the hikers have?

Tell why these are good snacks.

Name some good snacks to have at a class party.

Your Turn

At the Restaurant

Lisa and her family are eating in a restaurant. Lisa is not sure what to order. She likes everything on the menu. She can't make up her mind.

Help Lisa decide.
Choose a healthful meal for her.
Tell why you picked those foods.

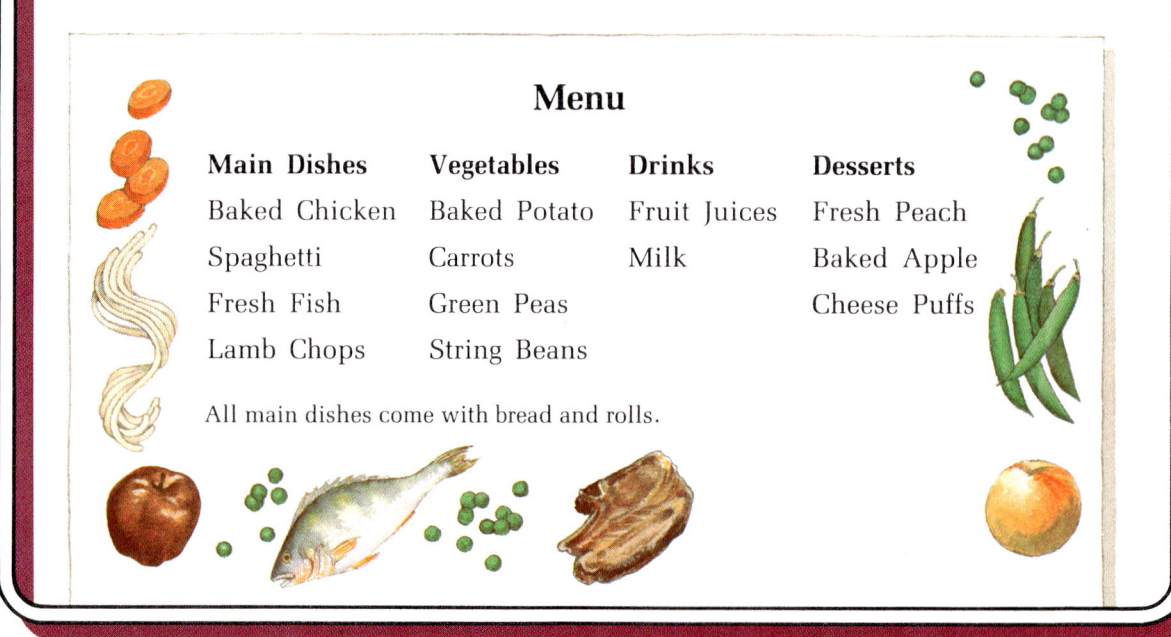

Menu

Main Dishes	Vegetables	Drinks	Desserts
Baked Chicken	Baked Potato	Fruit Juices	Fresh Peach
Spaghetti	Carrots	Milk	Baked Apple
Fresh Fish	Green Peas		Cheese Puffs
Lamb Chops	String Beans		

All main dishes come with bread and rolls.

Health in Action

1. Tell about a food. Don't say the name. Ask others to guess.

2. Look at the picture. Figure out the foods. Which gives you energy? Which helps you grow? Which is a vegetable?

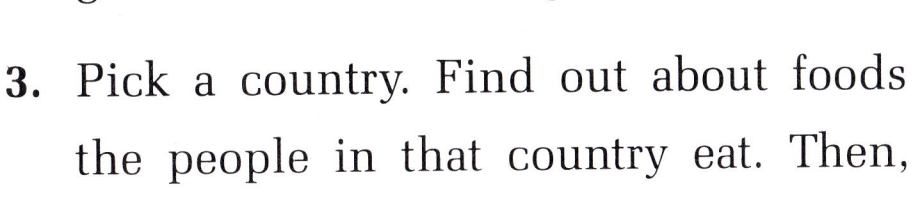

3. Pick a country. Find out about foods the people in that country eat. Then, tell the class what you have learned.

4. Read Joe's chart. How good is his diet? Can he make it better? Tell how.

racorts
adreb
sifh

Joe's Diet	
Breakfast	toast
Lunch	a pear
Dinner	fish
Snacks	milk

Do You Remember?

Your Health Words

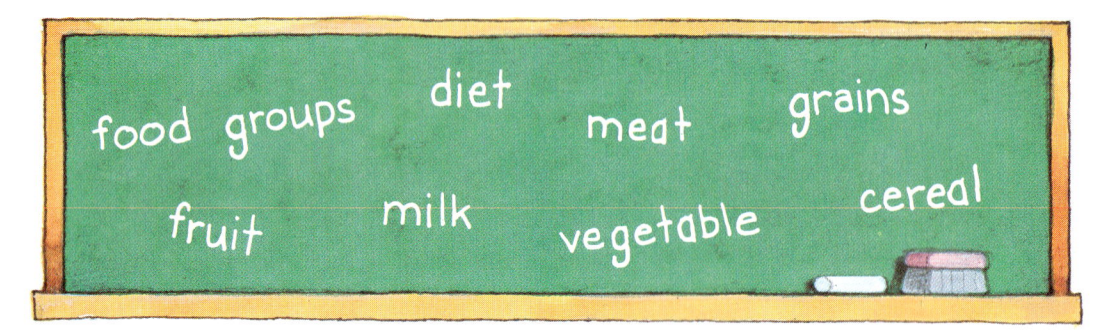

[chalkboard with words: food groups, diet, meat, grains, fruit, milk, vegetable, cereal]

Finish the sentences.

Use the Health Words.

1. Your ___ is made up of all the food you eat and drink.
2. There are four ___.
3. A good diet has ___ in it.

Your Health Ideas

1. Name the four food groups.
2. Tell what a good diet is.
3. Tell why a good diet is important.

Health Check-Up

Tell which sentences are true.

1. Apples and eggs are in the same food group.
2. Fruit is part of a good diet.
3. You should eat food from only one food group in a day.
4. Bread can take the place of vegetables.
5. Rice can take the place of bread.
6. Milk and cheese are in the same food group.
7. Beans can take the place of meat.
8. Meat does not help you grow.
9. Fruits and vegetables help you stay well.
10. Snacks can be part of your diet.

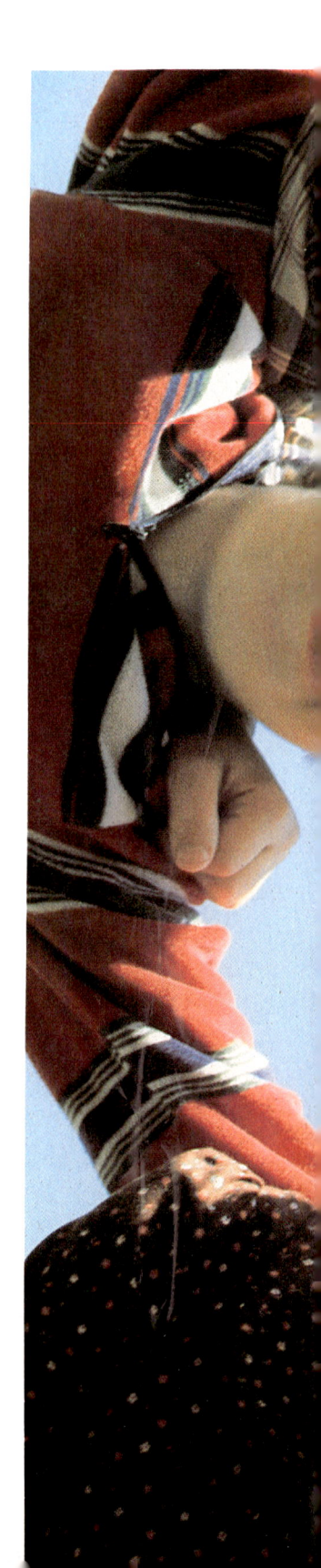

CHAPTER 4

Your Teeth

Help keep your smile healthy. Help take care of your teeth. Clean them after eating. Eat fewer sweets. Protect your teeth from injury. Get regular check-ups. Your teeth are an important part of you. You should have them for a long time. Take care of them every day.

What can you do to take care of your teeth every day?

Health Words

primary teeth   dentists
permanent teeth   brush
molars   floss
crown   decay

67

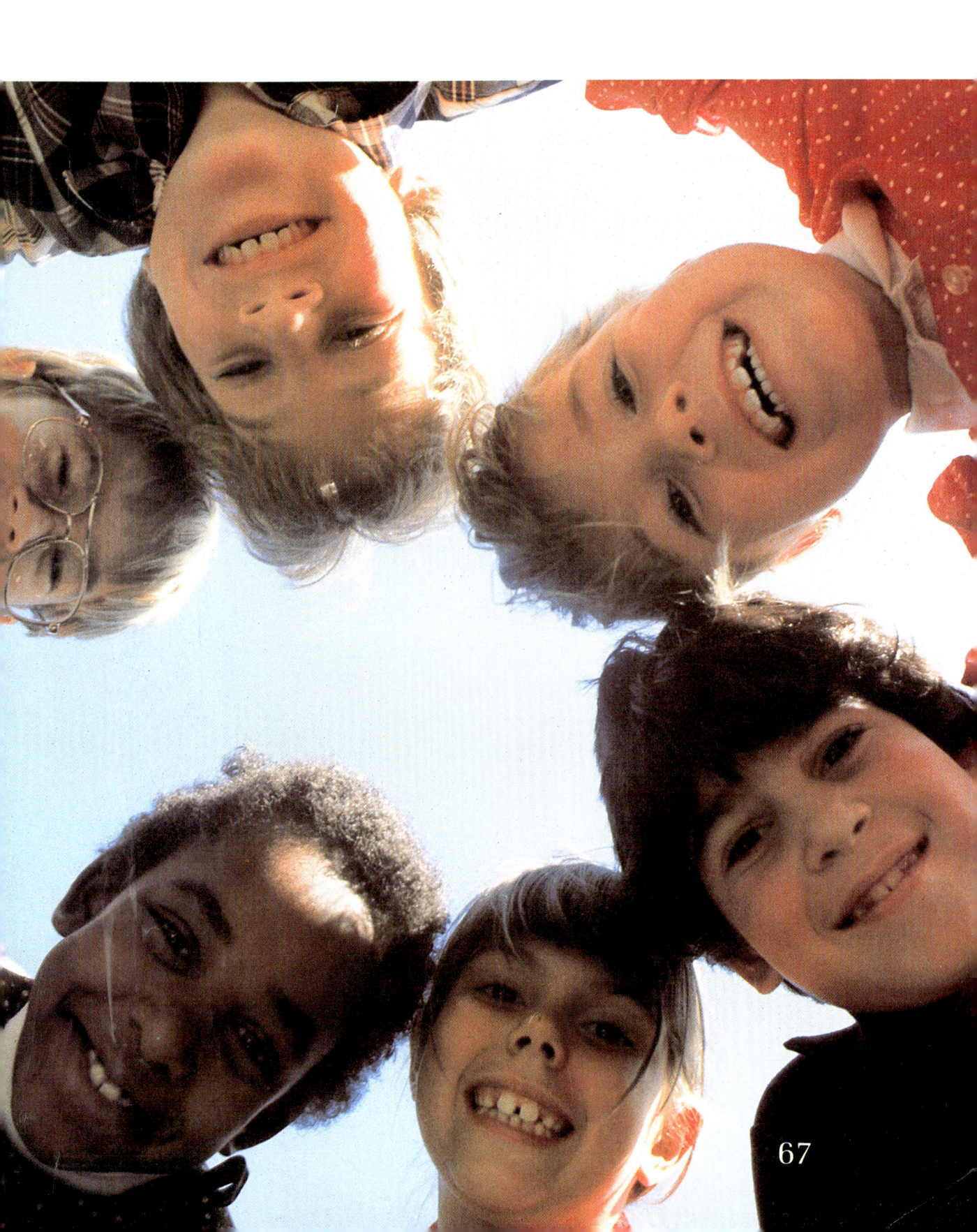

Teeth You Lose and Teeth You Keep

Your first teeth are called primary teeth. There are 20 in all. They are the teeth you lose. Permanent teeth take their place. There are 32 permanent teeth. Six-year molars are the first.

Take care of all your teeth. Having healthy primary teeth is important. It can help give permanent teeth a healthy start.

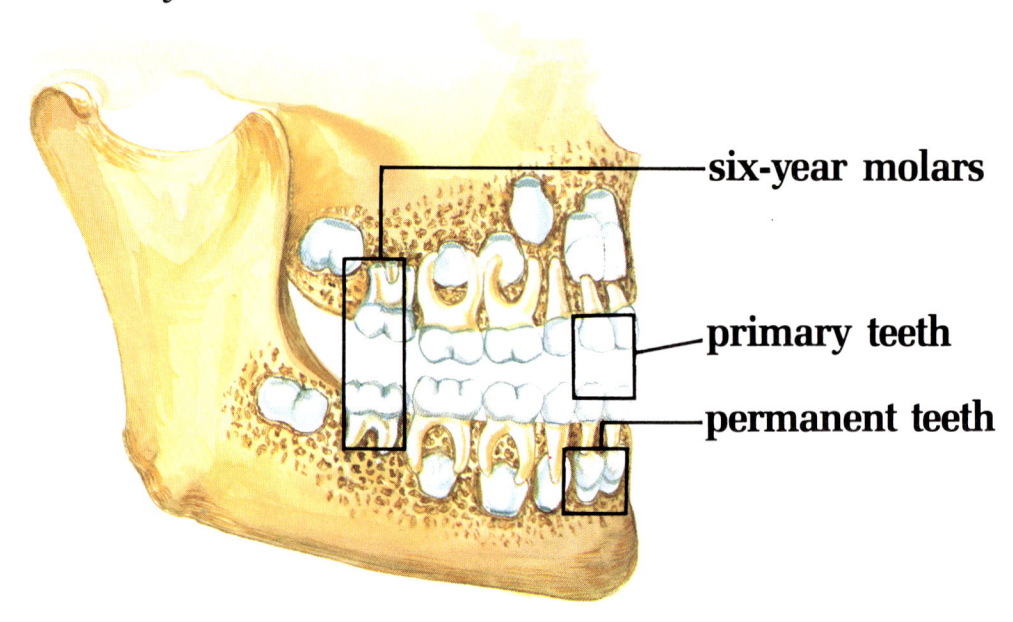

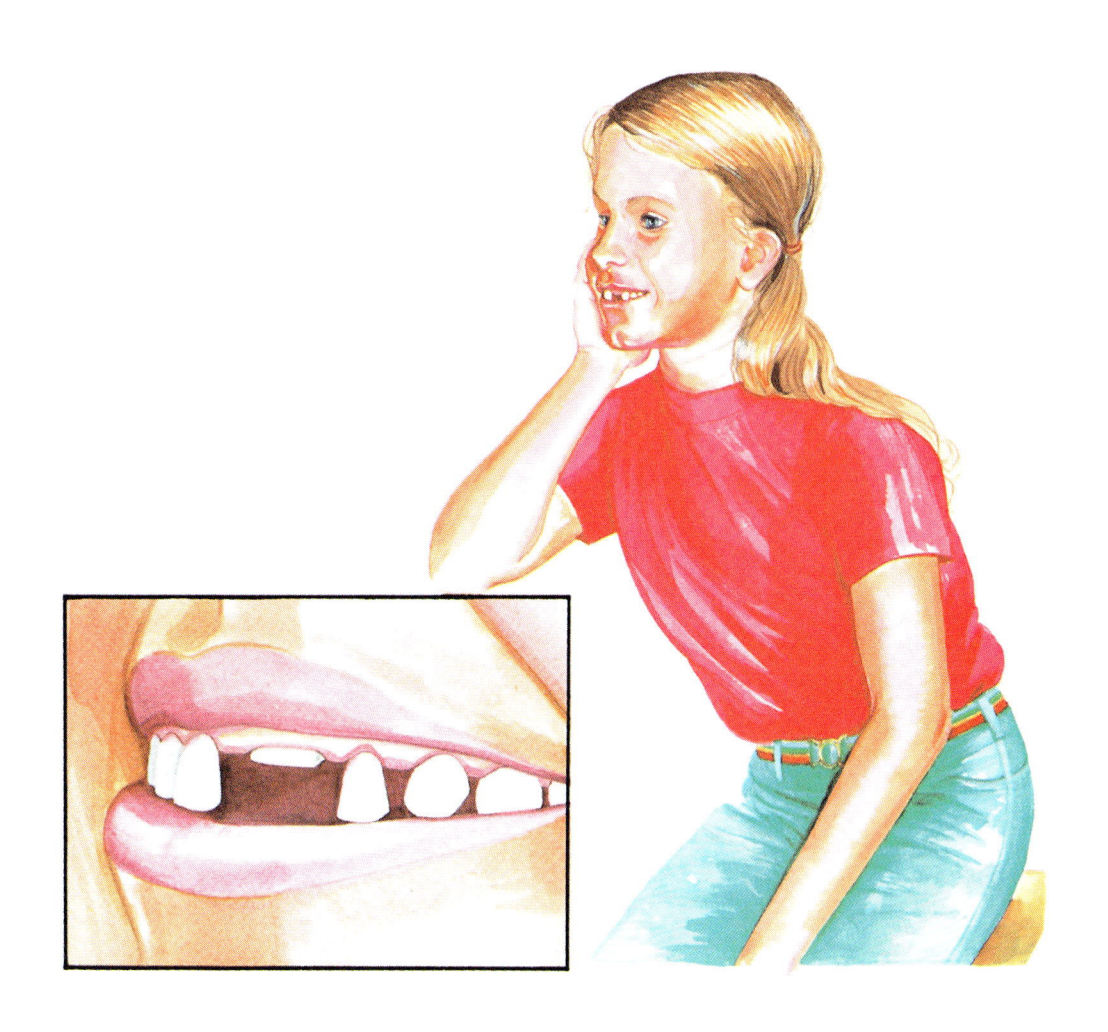

Look at the teeth on page 68.

Point to the primary teeth.

Find the permanent teeth.

Point to the six-year molars.

Look at the girl's teeth.

She has primary and permanent teeth.

Why is it important for her to take care of all her primary teeth?

Parts of a Tooth

Look at your teeth in a mirror. What you see are the crowns. The crowns help you bite or chew food.

Most of each tooth is hidden under the gum. The hidden part is called the root. It helps hold the tooth in place.

Take care of your teeth. Brush them every day.

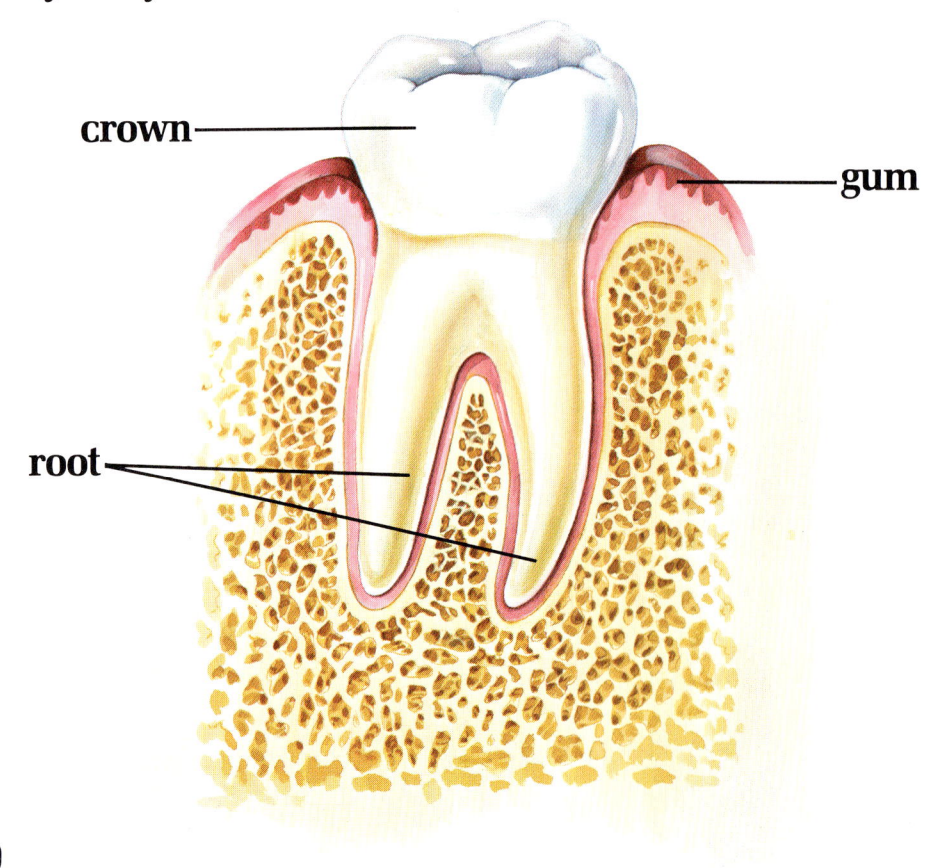

crown

gum

root

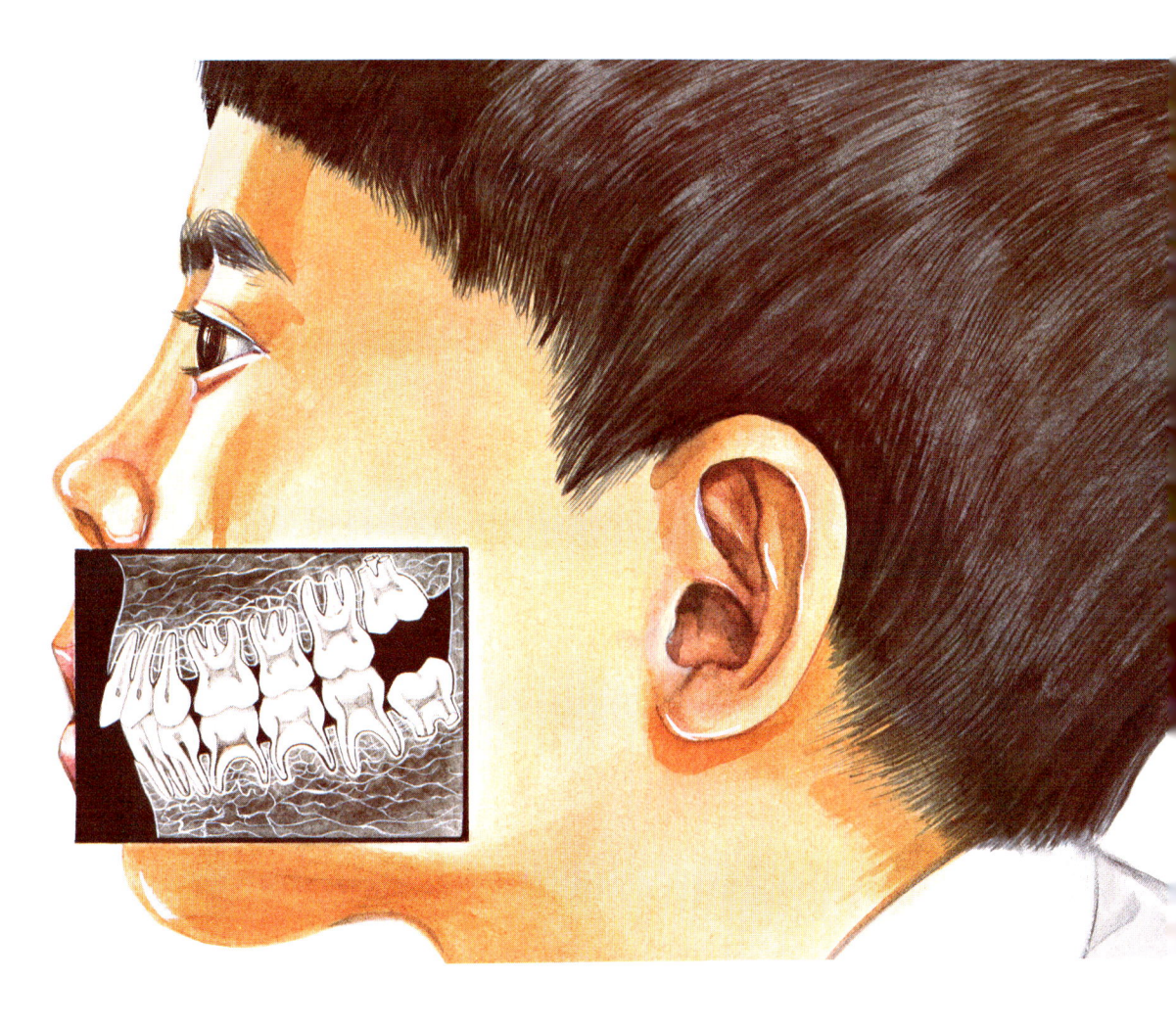

Look at both pictures.

Point to a root and a crown.

Point to the gums.

Use your tongue.

Rub the crowns of your teeth.

What do they feel like?

How can you take care of them?

Taking Care of Your Teeth

You can help take care of your teeth. You can help keep them clean. Cleaning your teeth helps keep them healthy. Cleaning helps stop tooth decay. Not eating sweets between meals helps, too.

Brush your teeth after you eat. Brush before bedtime, too. Floss to clean between teeth. Help keep your teeth healthy.

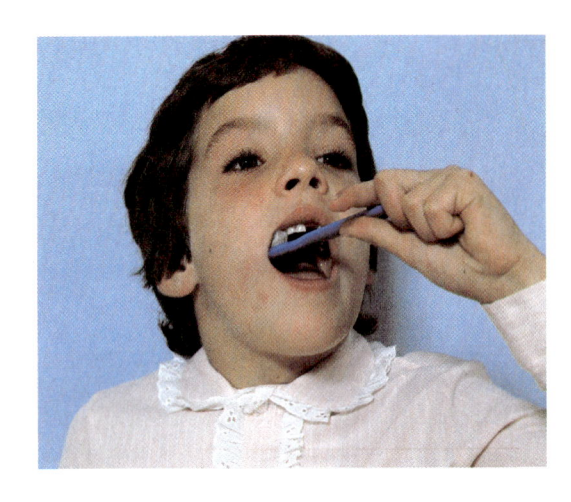

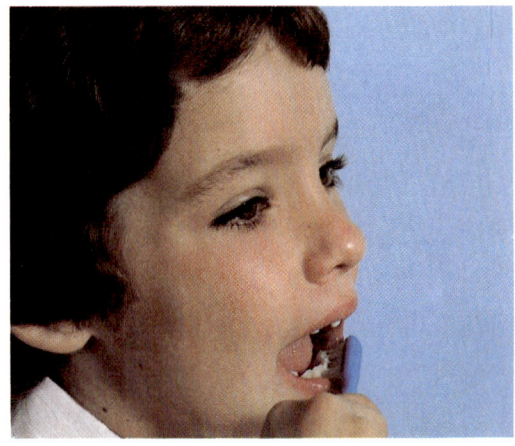

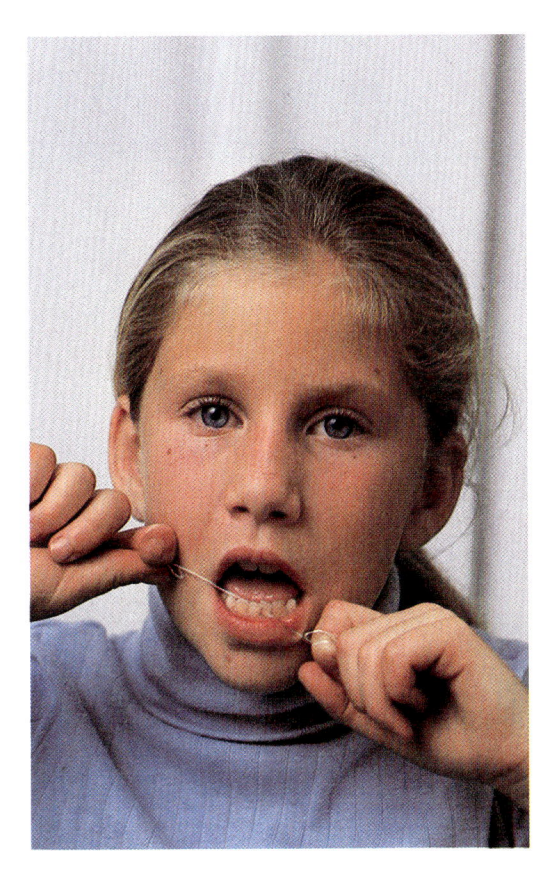

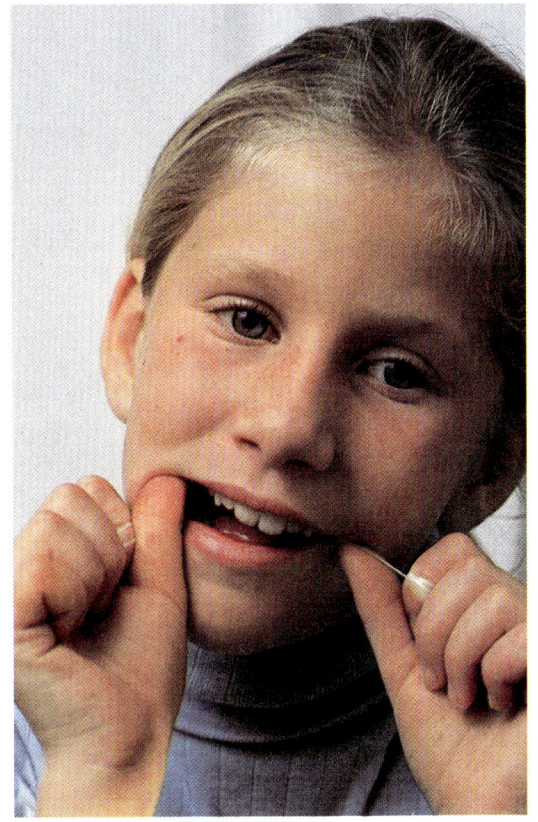

Look at the pictures on page 72.
Tell how to brush your teeth.

Look at the pictures on this page.
Tell how to floss your teeth.

How does flossing help keep teeth clean?

Why is it important to brush and floss your teeth?

Health Highlight

A Toothbrush Is Born

Long ago, people used rags to clean their teeth. They put chalk on a rag and rubbed it on their teeth.

In 1770, a man named William Addis came up with an idea. He made little holes in one end of a meat bone. He put bristles into the holes. A toothbrush was born.

Why does a toothbrush clean teeth better than a rag?

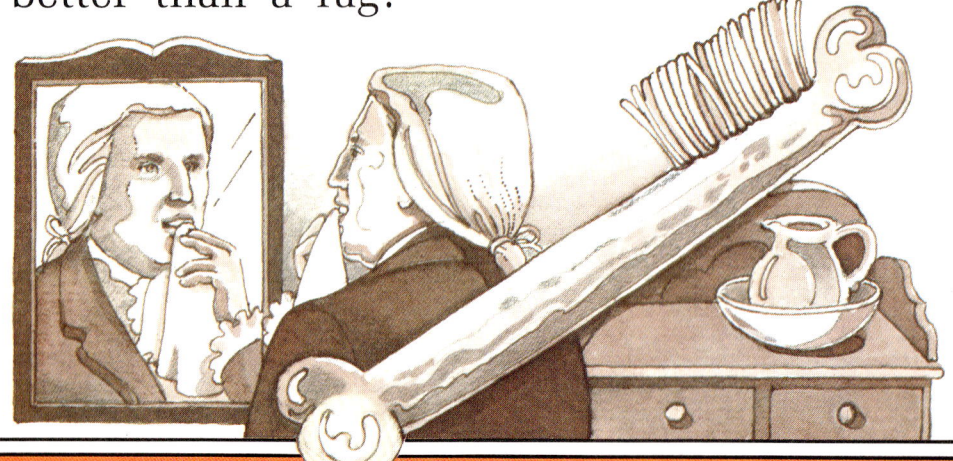

Going, Seeing, and Doing

1. Go into your bathroom. Which of these things do you have? How often should you use them?

2. Look at your teeth in a mirror. How many primary teeth do you have? How many have you lost? How many permanent teeth do you have coming in?

3. Show how to floss your teeth. Ask for help, if you need it. Then, tell how flossing can help your teeth.

Getting Help for Your Teeth

What do you know about your teeth? Do they fit together? Is there tooth decay? Are your permanent teeth growing the way they should be? Are your gums healthy?

Dentists can find the answers to these questions. They can help you keep your teeth healthy.

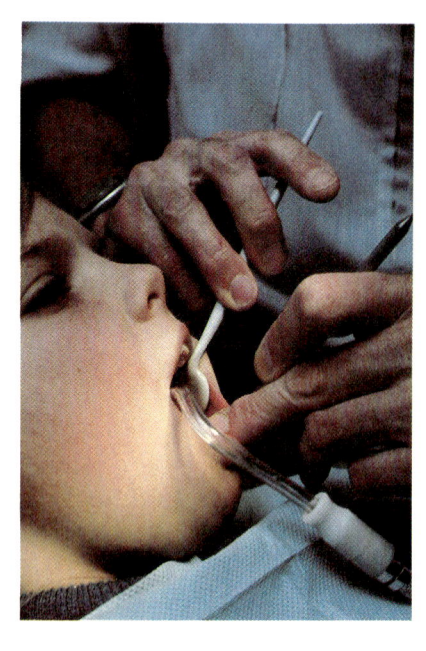

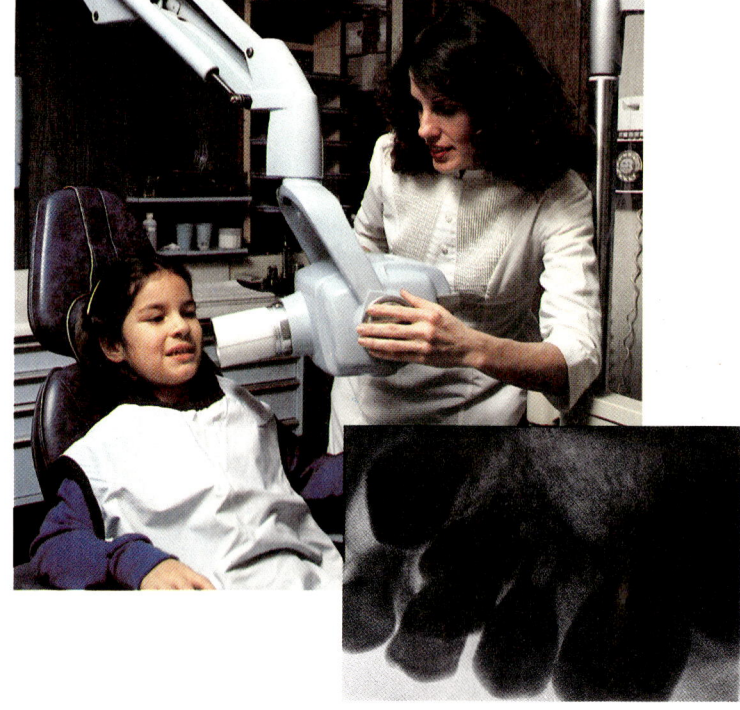

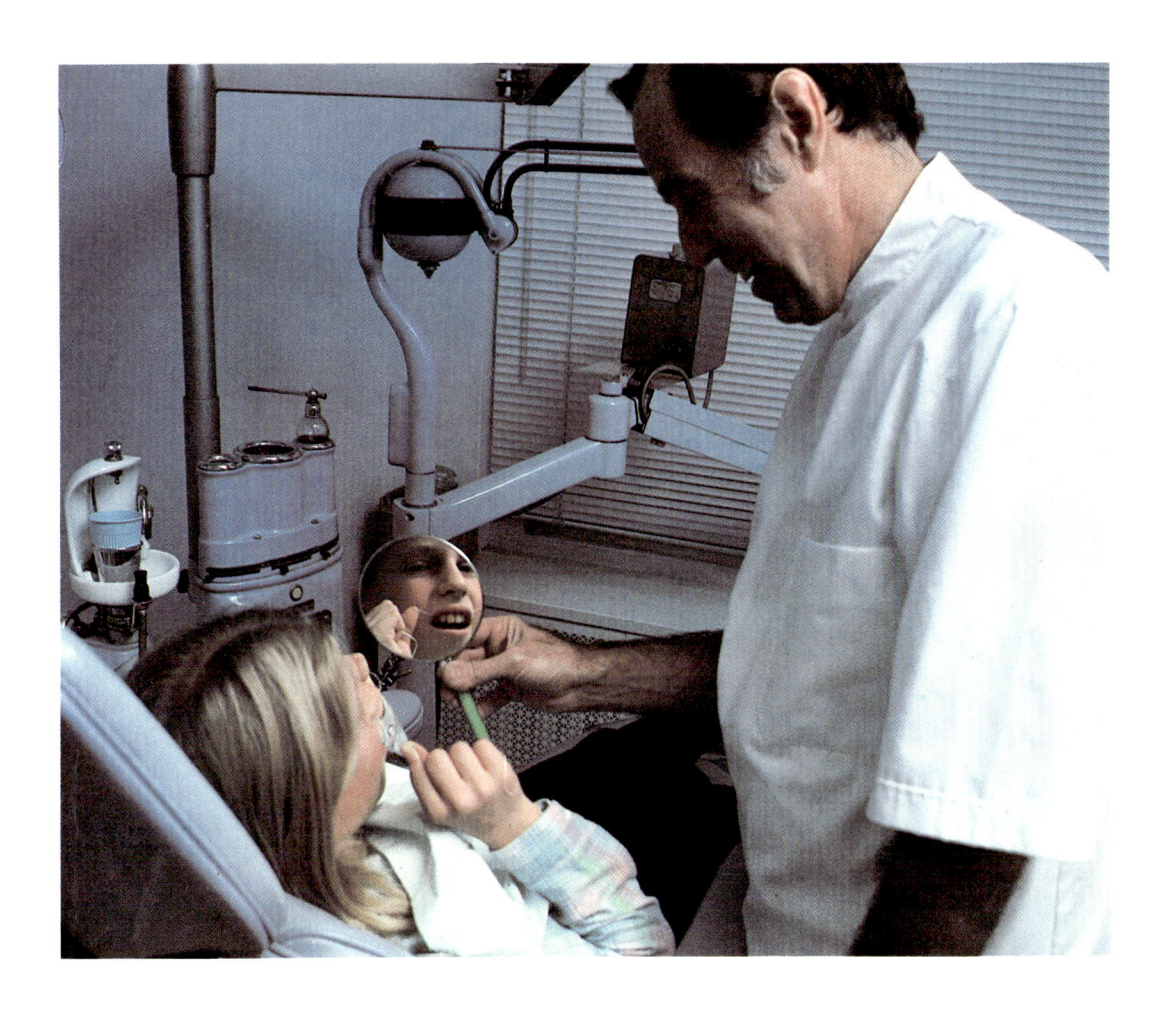

Look at the pictures on page 76.
What are the dentists doing?

Look at the picture on this page.
What is the girl learning?

In what other ways can a dentist help you?

What can you do to help?

Protecting Your Teeth from Injury

Your teeth can get chipped or broken. You can help protect them, though. Wait your turn at water fountains. Keep pencils out of your mouth. Follow safety rules.

You need your teeth. They help you eat. They help you talk. They help you look and feel good. Keep them safe.

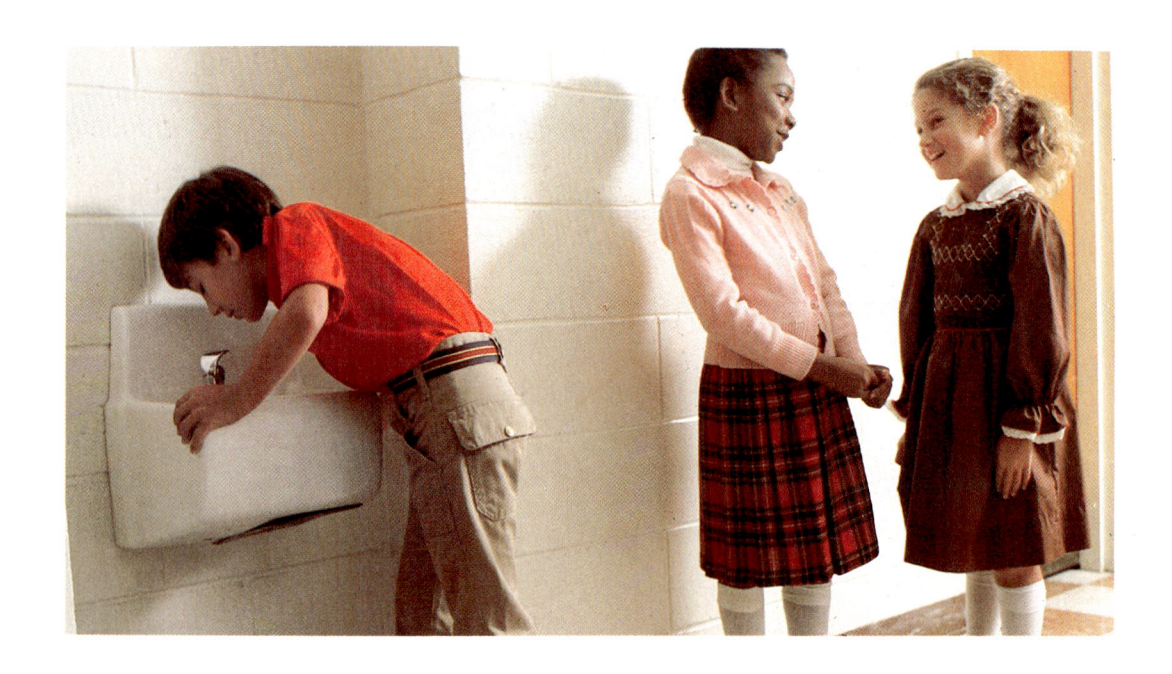

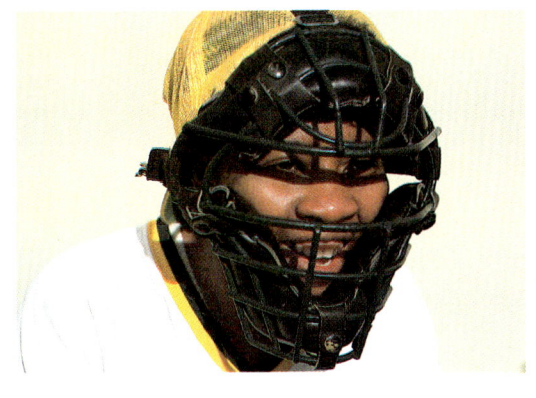

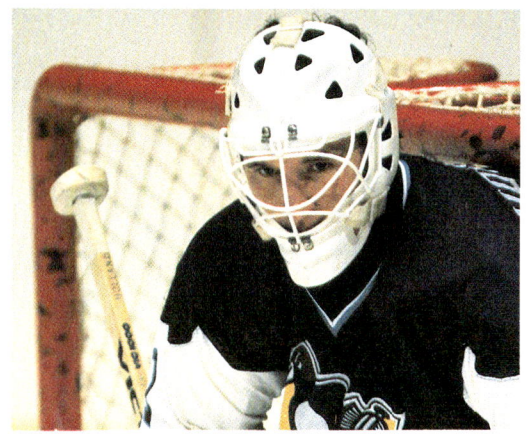

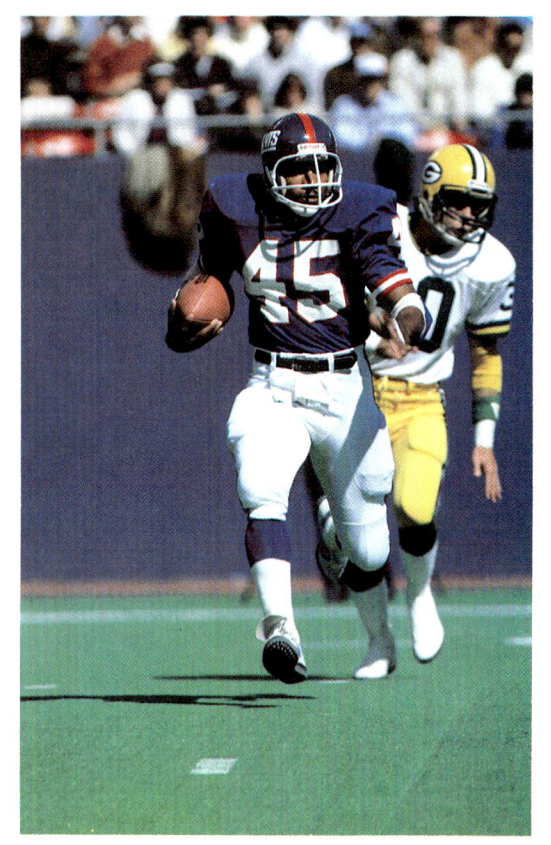

Look at the children on page 78.

How are they helping to protect their teeth?

Look at the other pictures.

How are the teeth protected?

Tell other ways to help protect your teeth from injury.

Why should you protect your teeth?

79

Your Turn

No Toothbrush

Lois is sleeping at a friend's house. She brought her floss, but she forgot her toothbrush. It was the first time something like that had happened. Lois wants to clean her teeth. She does not want to use her friend's toothbrush.

Help Lois.

Tell how she can clean her teeth this one time without a toothbrush.

Tell why your ideas would help.

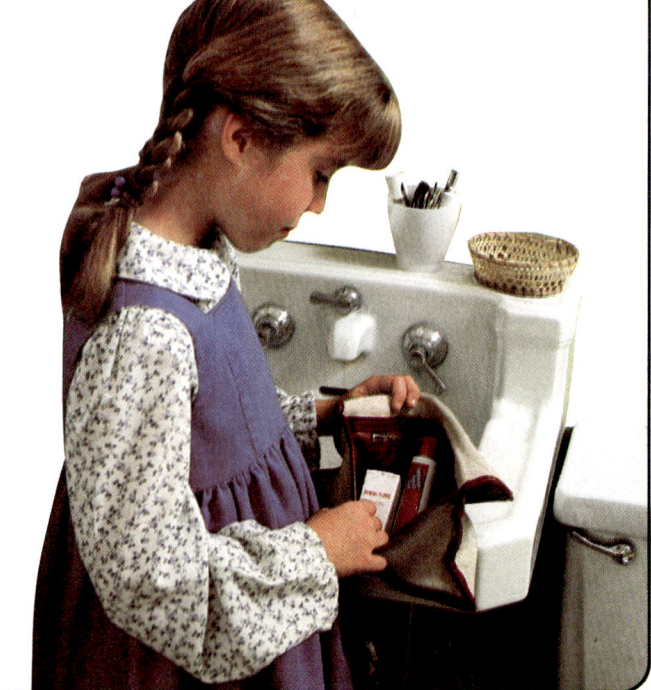

Health in Action

1. Trace this picture of a tooth. Draw a line where the gum starts. Color the root. Write the word *Crown* next to the crown.

2. Write questions to ask the dentist. Give them to the dentist at your next check-up.

3. Each row of words can make a sentence. The sentences tell about ways to help your teeth. What are they? Write them the right way. Use your own paper.

   after Brush eating.
   dentist the Visit.
   teeth your Protect.

4. Make a list. Tell ways to protect teeth from injury.

Do You Remember?

Your Health Words

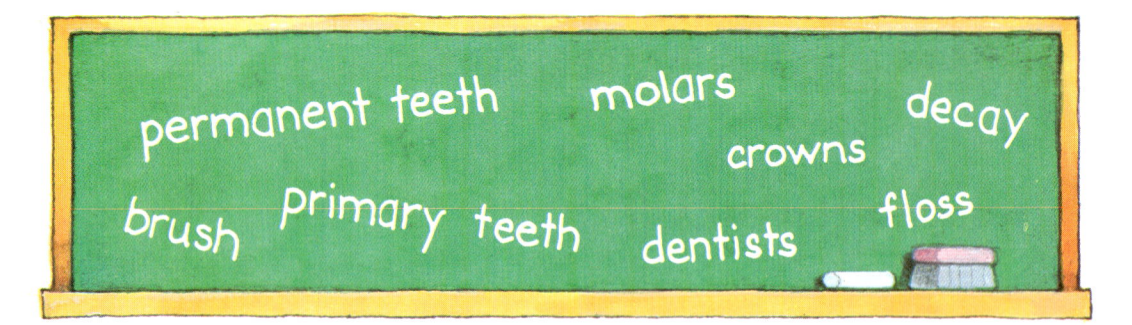

permanent teeth   molars   decay
crowns
brush   primary teeth   dentists   floss

Answer the questions.

Use the Health Words.

1. Who should check your teeth?
2. How can you clean your teeth?
3. What part of your teeth do you brush?

Your Health Ideas

1. Tell how a dentist helps your teeth.
2. Tell how to brush your teeth.
3. Tell how to help keep your teeth safe.

Health Check-Up

Tell which sentences are true.

1. Your gums are part of your teeth.
2. Your first teeth are called permanent teeth.
3. You can see the crown of a tooth.
4. You can help keep your teeth clean.
5. You should brush your teeth before eating.
6. Dentists check for tooth decay.
7. You can clean between your teeth.
8. It is safe to put pencils in your mouth.
9. Your teeth help you chew food.
10. Teeth can never get chipped.

CHAPTER 5

Taking Care of Your Health

Your body is very special. The more you know about it, the more you will know about your health. Learn about your body. Learn about ways to help keep it well. Taking care of your body is taking care of your health.

How can you help take care of your health?

Health Words

germs   doctors
cough   check-up
sneeze   vision
nurses

85

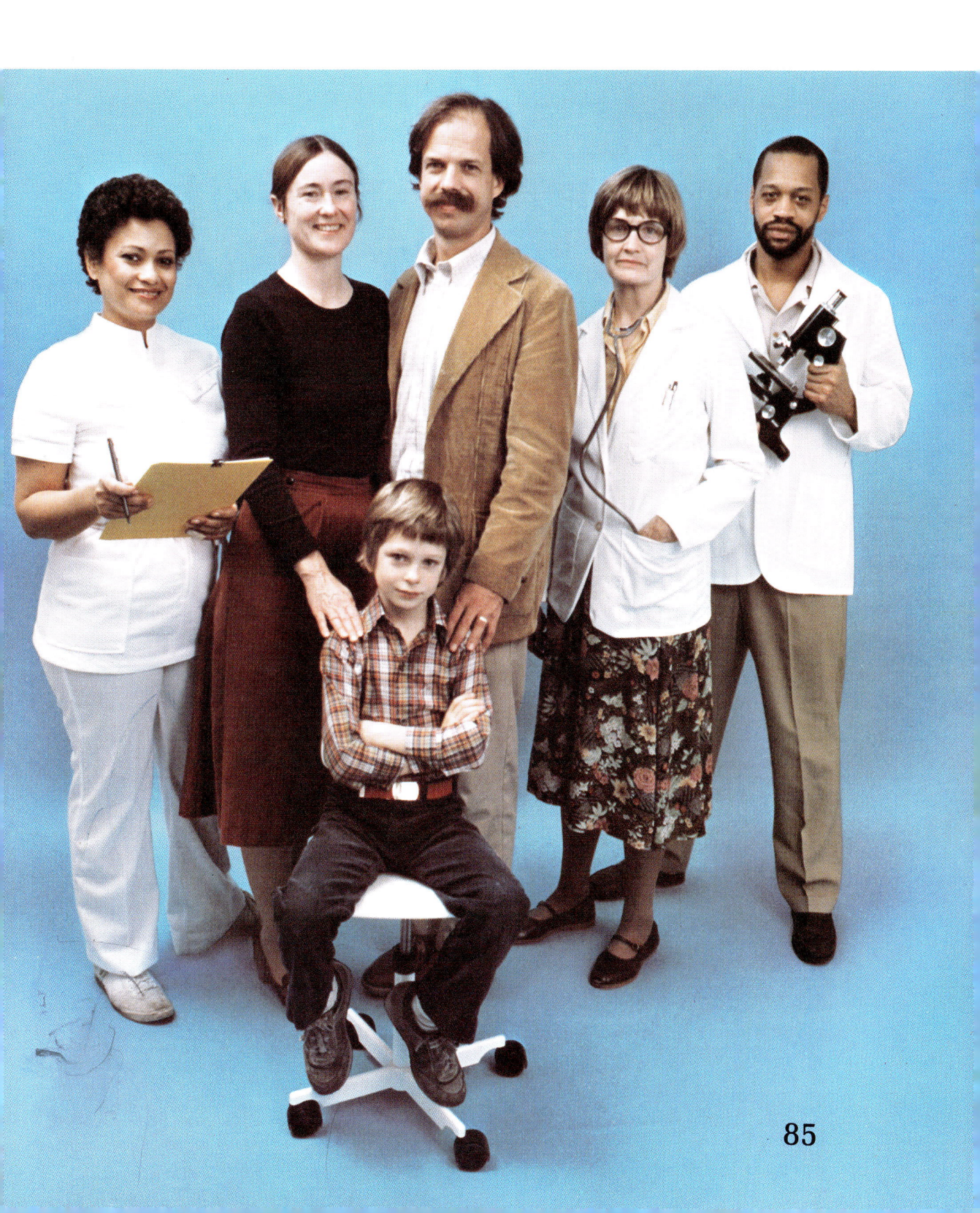

Knowing About Germs

Germs are living things. They live everywhere. They are in the air, on the ground, and in the water. Germs are very tiny. You need a microscope to see them.

Most germs are harmless, but some are not. Some germs that get inside your body can make you ill.

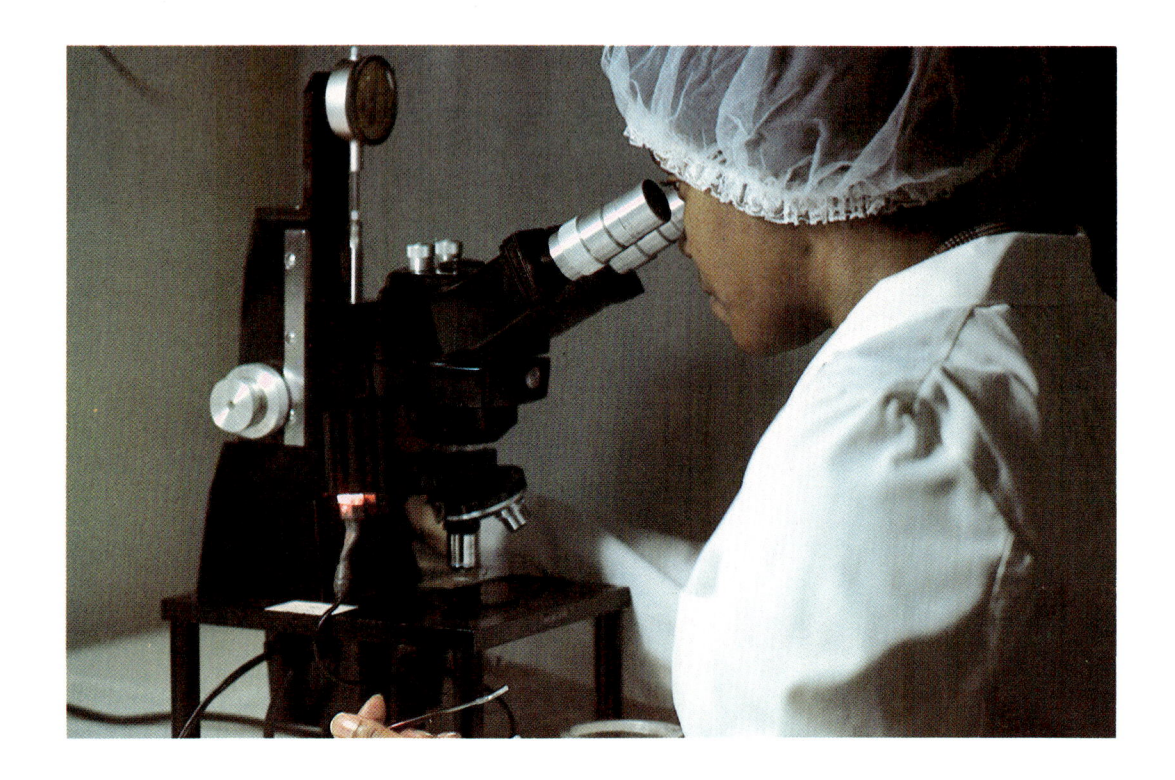

microscope

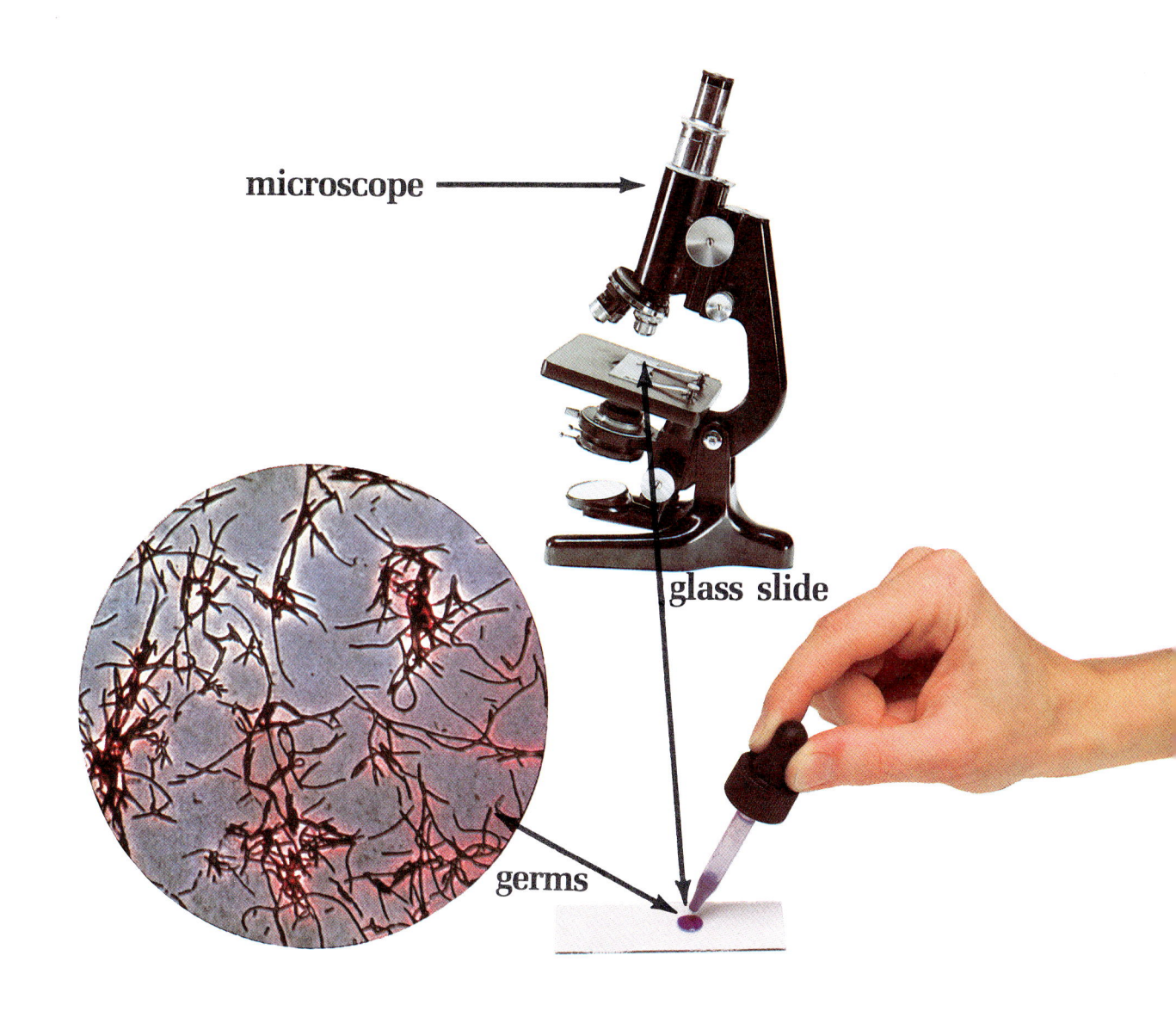

glass slide

germs

Look at the pictures on this page.
Point to the germs.
Where might they be found?
Can you see germs in these places?
Tell why.

Germs Can Spread

Germs live inside everyone. When you cough or sneeze, the germs inside you spread into the air. Germs can also spread from your mouth to your glass. They can spread to your food.

Cover your mouth when you sneeze or cough. Don't share drinks from the same glass. Do your part to help keep germs from spreading.

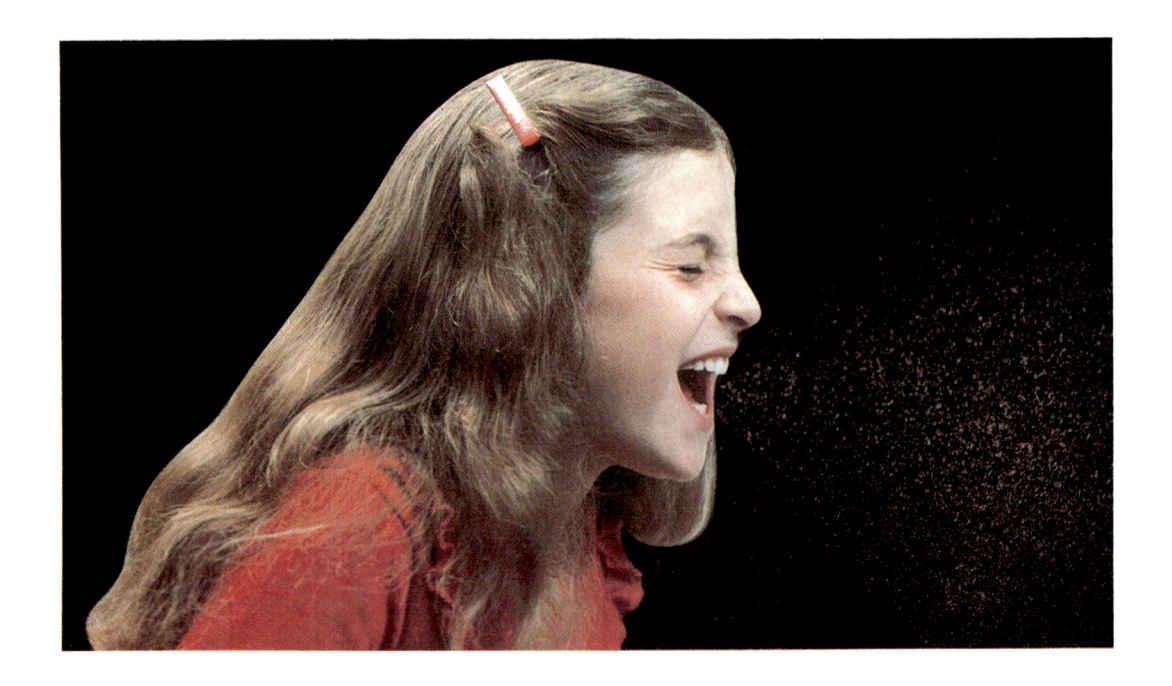

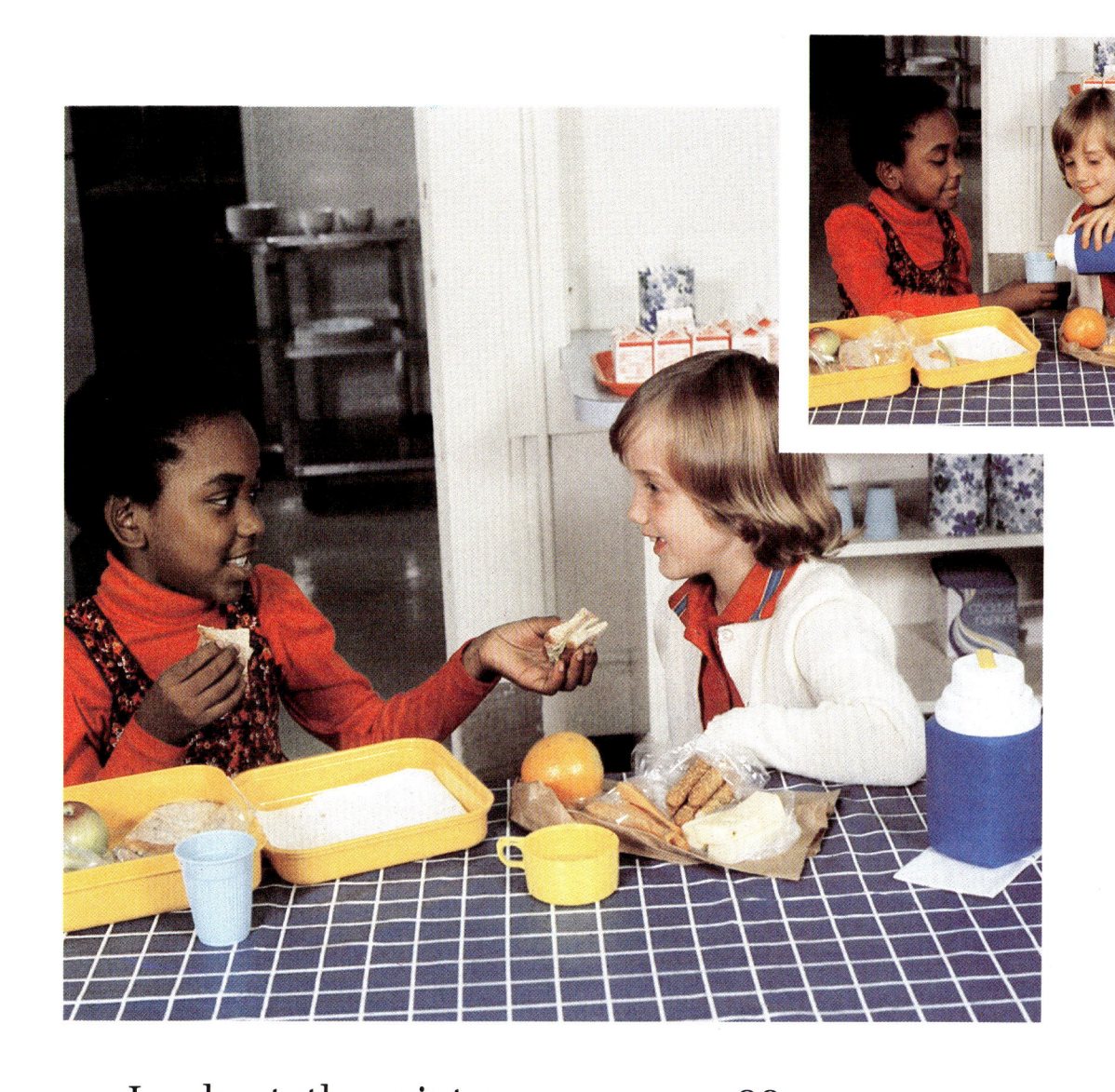

Look at the picture on page 88.

How is the girl helping to spread germs?

Look at the pictures on this page.

How are the girls sharing food?

How are they helping to stop the spread of germs?

Sometimes You May Feel Ill

There may be times when you do not feel well. Some part of your body may hurt. Your nose may be stuffed up. These are some ways your body tells you something is wrong.

When you do not feel well, tell your teacher or the school nurse. Tell a grown-up in your family.

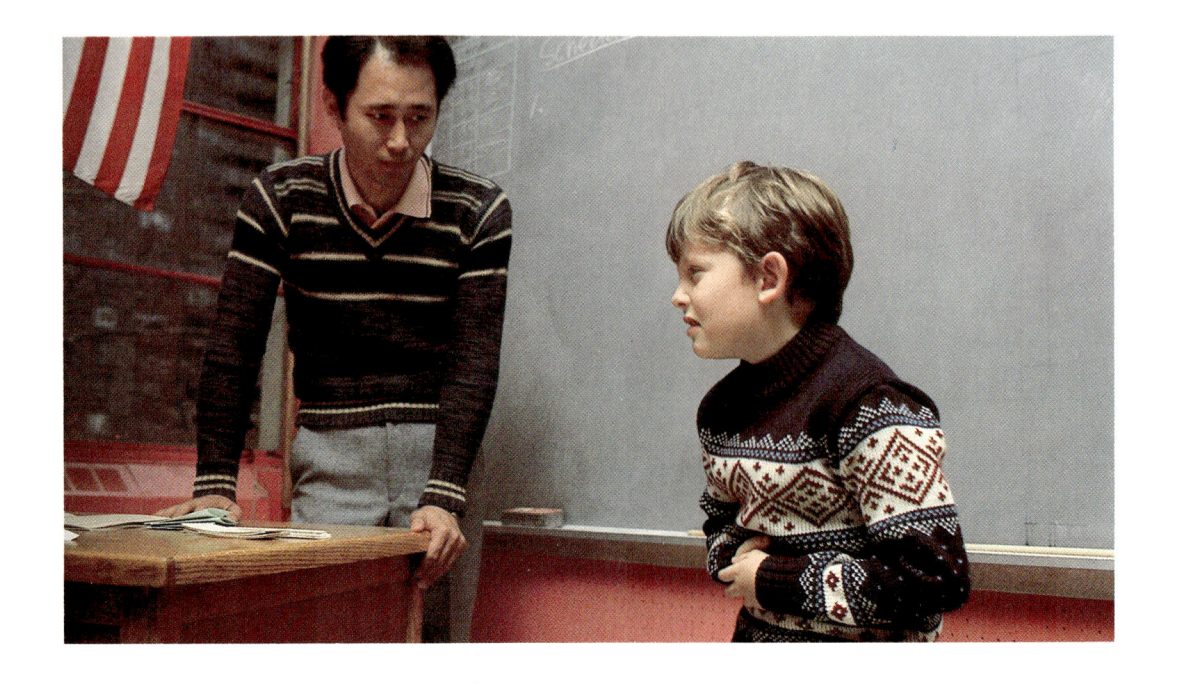

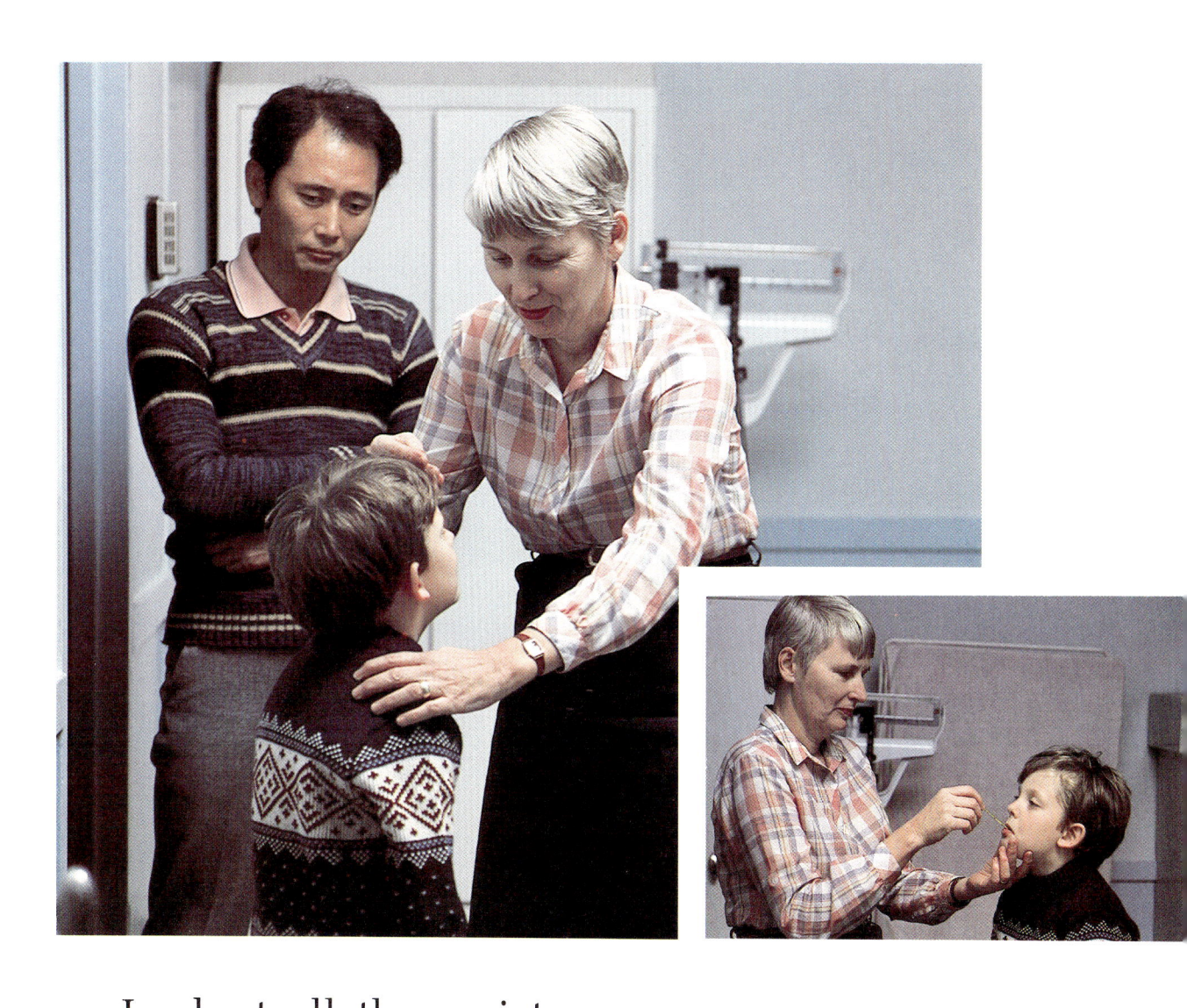

Look at all three pictures.

How is the boy feeling?

Whom did he tell?

Why was this a good thing to do?

How else could he get the help he might need?

A Cold Is Not Something to Share

You can help keep cold germs from spreading. Stay home when you have a cold. Throw away the tissues you use. Get plenty of rest and sleep. Drink a lot of water and juices. Get well. Getting well is the best way to keep cold germs from spreading.

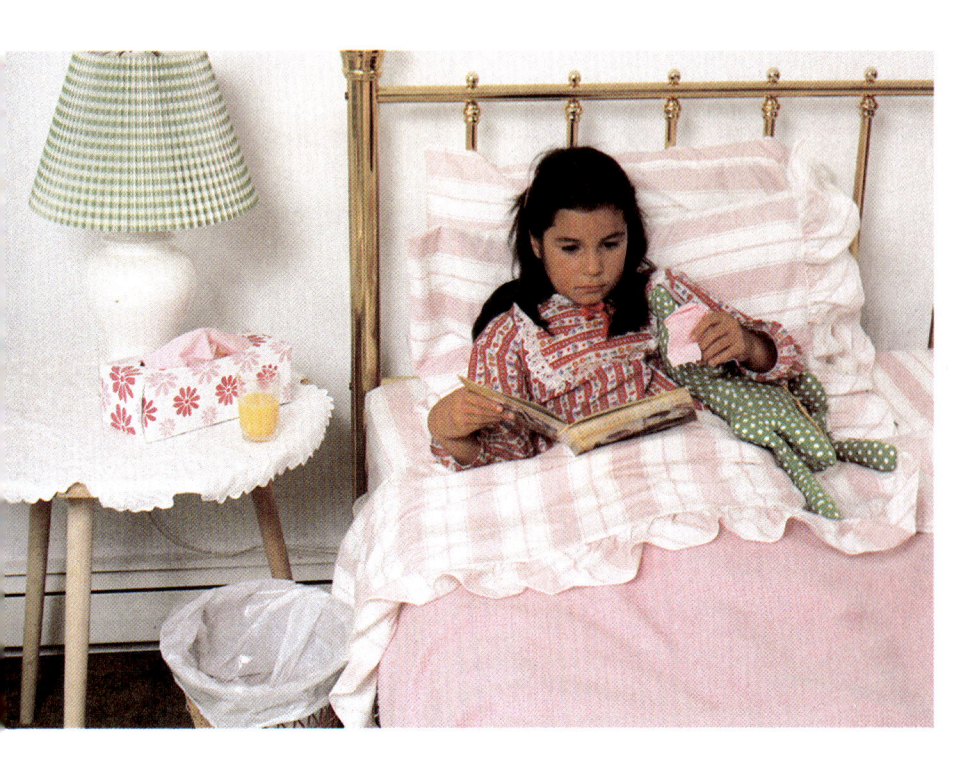

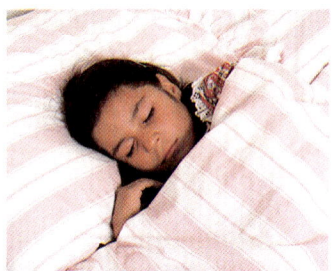

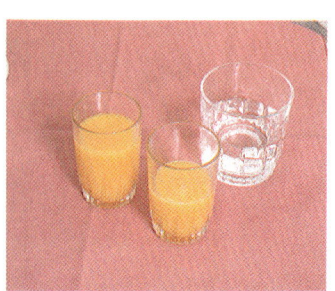

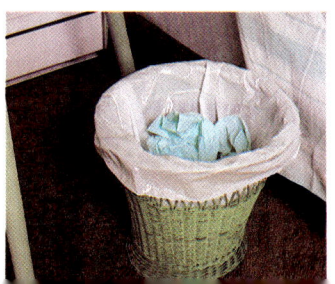

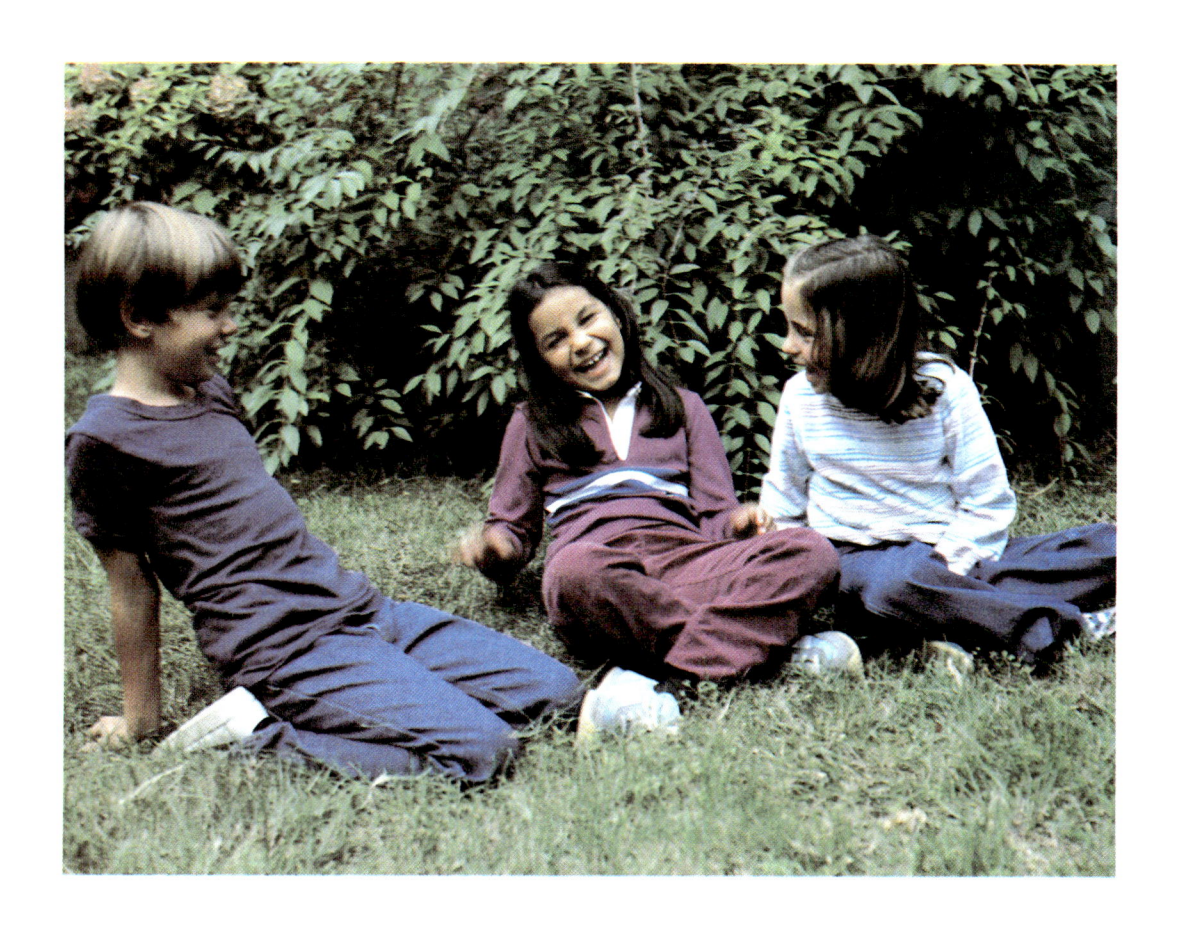

Look at the pictures on page 92.

How is the girl helping to take care of her cold?

How is she helping others stay well?

Look at the picture on this page.

How do you know the girl is better?

Why is it important to stay home with a cold?

The Doctor Looks

What do you know about your body? How tall are you? Are you growing the way you should? Are your eyes and ears healthy?

Doctors can give you a check-up. They can find answers to these kinds of questions. The answers help them learn about your health. They help you learn about it, too.

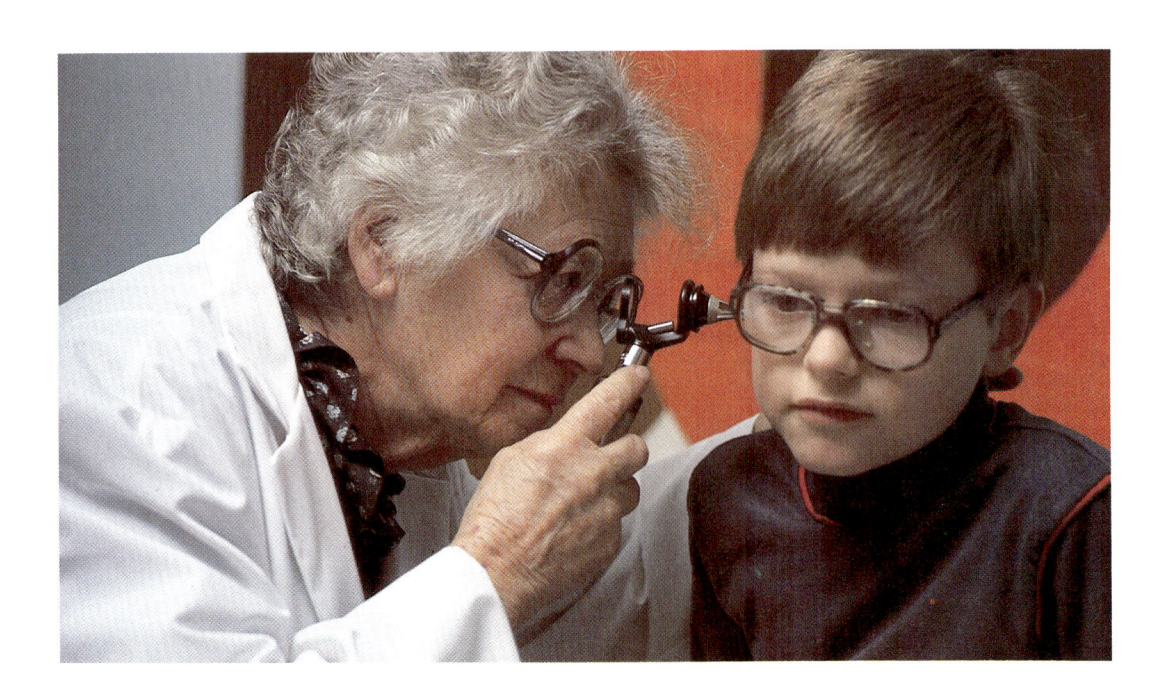

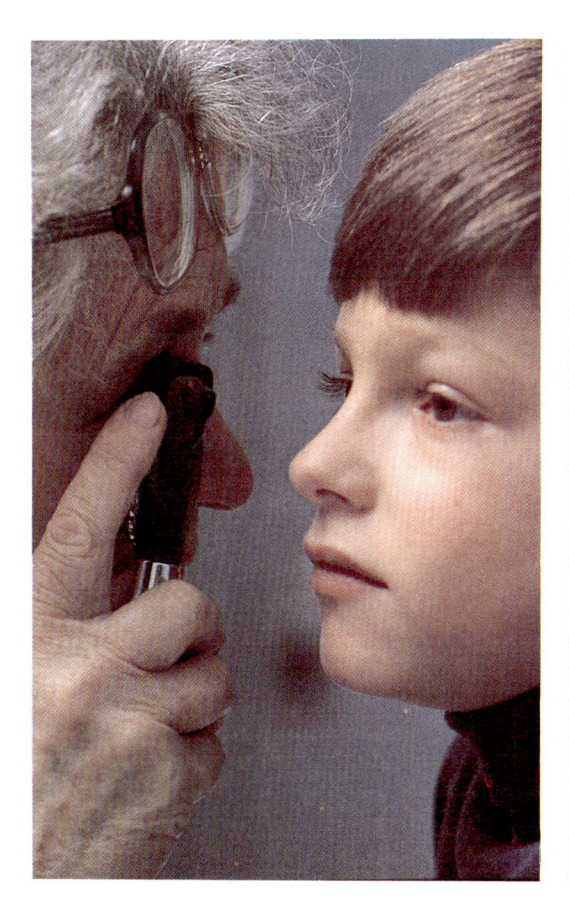

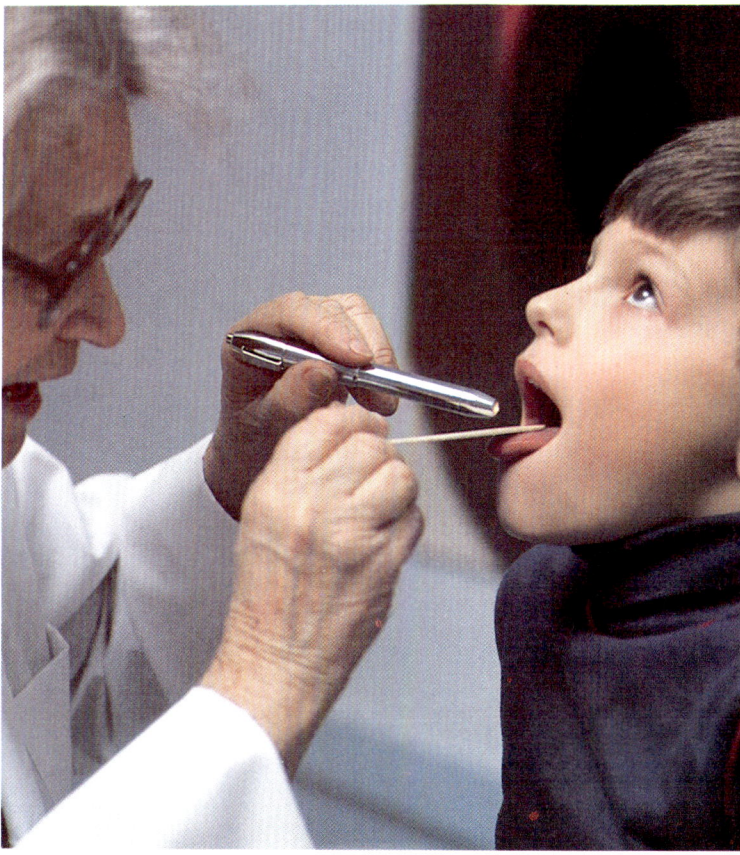

Look at all three pictures.

What is the doctor doing?

What is the doctor finding out about the boy?

What else can she find out?

What will the boy learn about himself?

Why is it important to learn about these things?

Wearing Glasses

An eye test may be part of a check-up. The test helps the doctor find out if you need glasses. Many people wear glasses. Without them their vision may be fuzzy.

If your vision seems fuzzy, tell a grown-up in your family. Tell your teacher. Get the help you may need to see your world at its best.

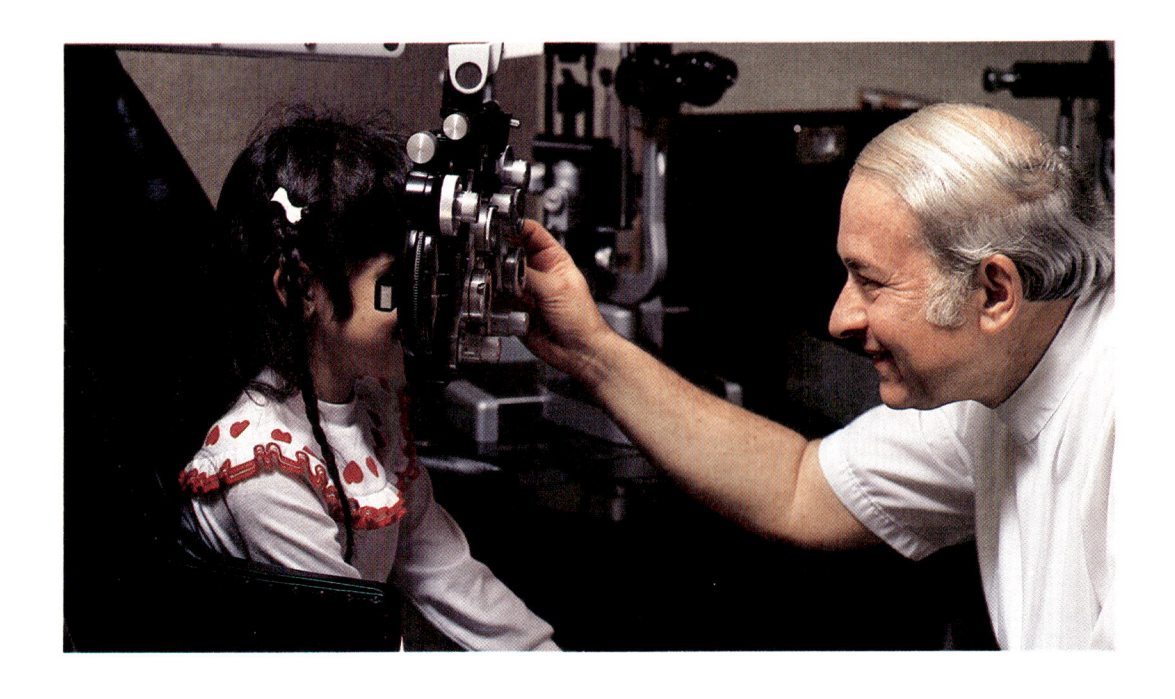

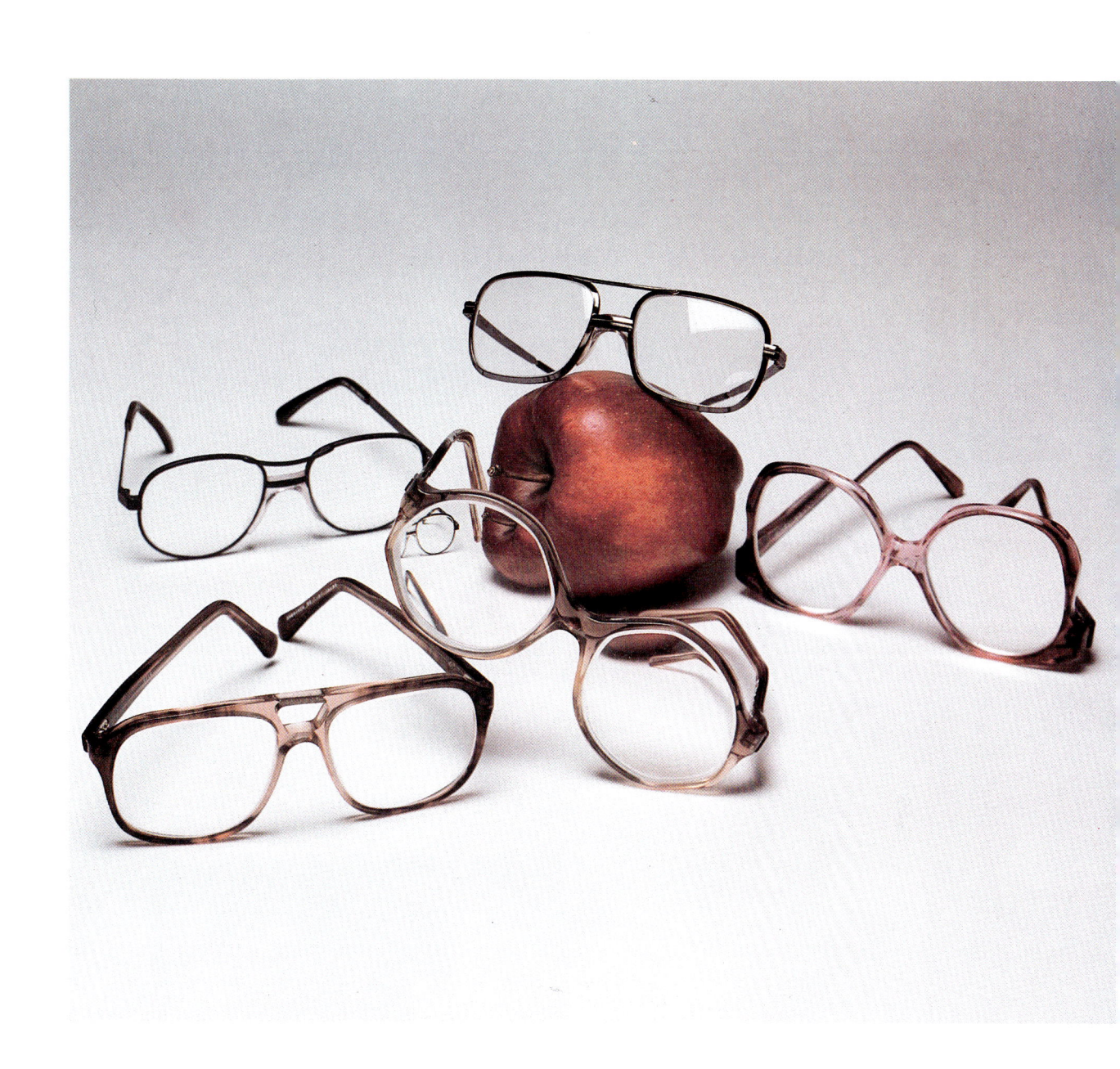

Look at the picture on page 96.
What is the girl doing?
Why is an eye test important?
How do glasses help some people?

Health Highlight

A Machine that Sees and Talks

This is a brand new machine. It helps people who can't see.

The machine has many parts. One part takes pictures. Another part looks at the pictures and speaks. It tells about what is ahead. It tells how far away things are.

How can the machine help someone who can't see?

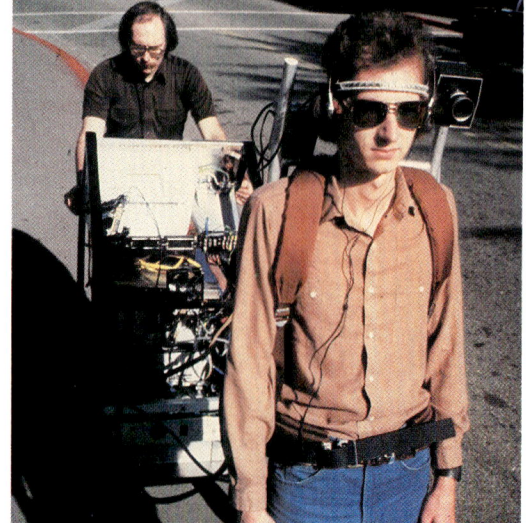

Going, Seeing, and Doing

1. Share a drink with a friend. Share the drink in a healthful way. Tell why your way of sharing was healthful.

2. Watch people who are sharing something to drink. Are they helping to spread germs? Are they helping to keep germs from spreading? How do you know?

3. Make a list. Tell some ways to take care of a cold.

The Doctor Listens

There are many things to learn about your body. Your heart pumps blood. Your lungs help you breathe. Be sure your heart and lungs are healthy. Have a doctor listen to them. Learn about all the parts of your body. Get regular check-ups.

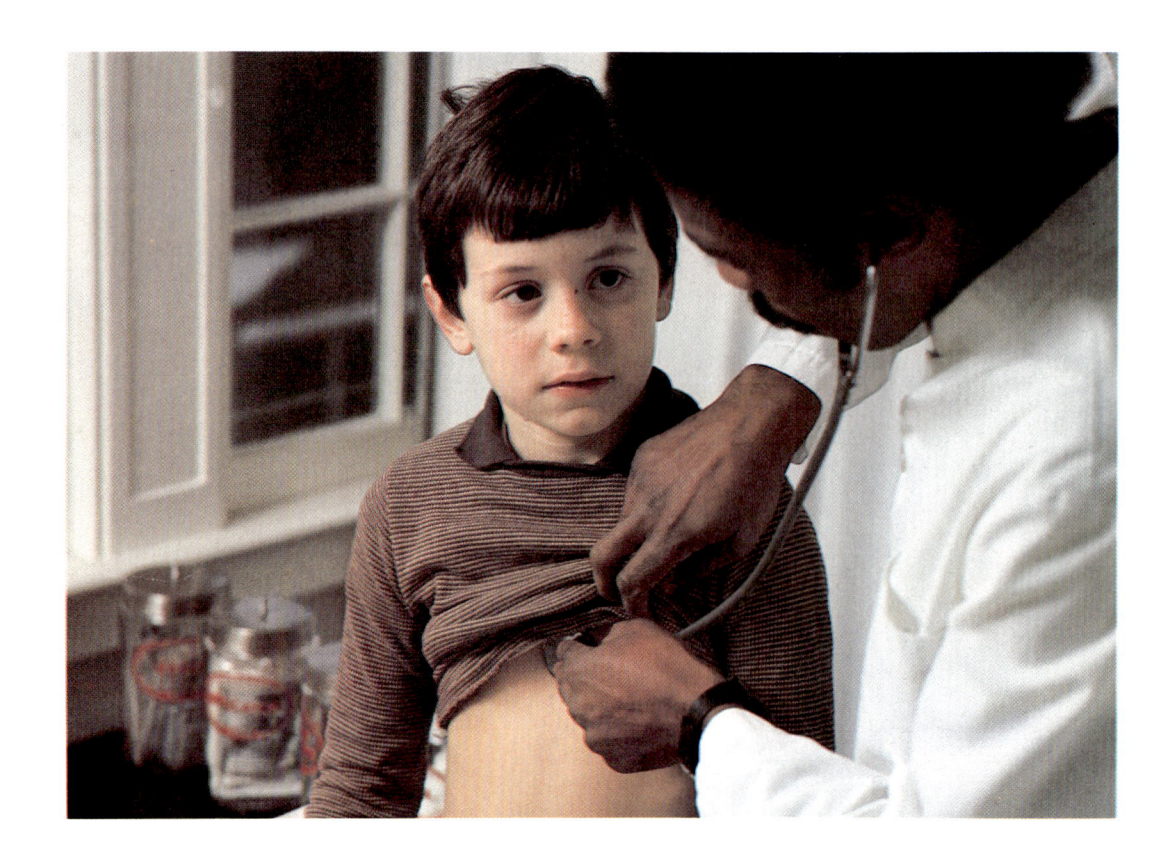

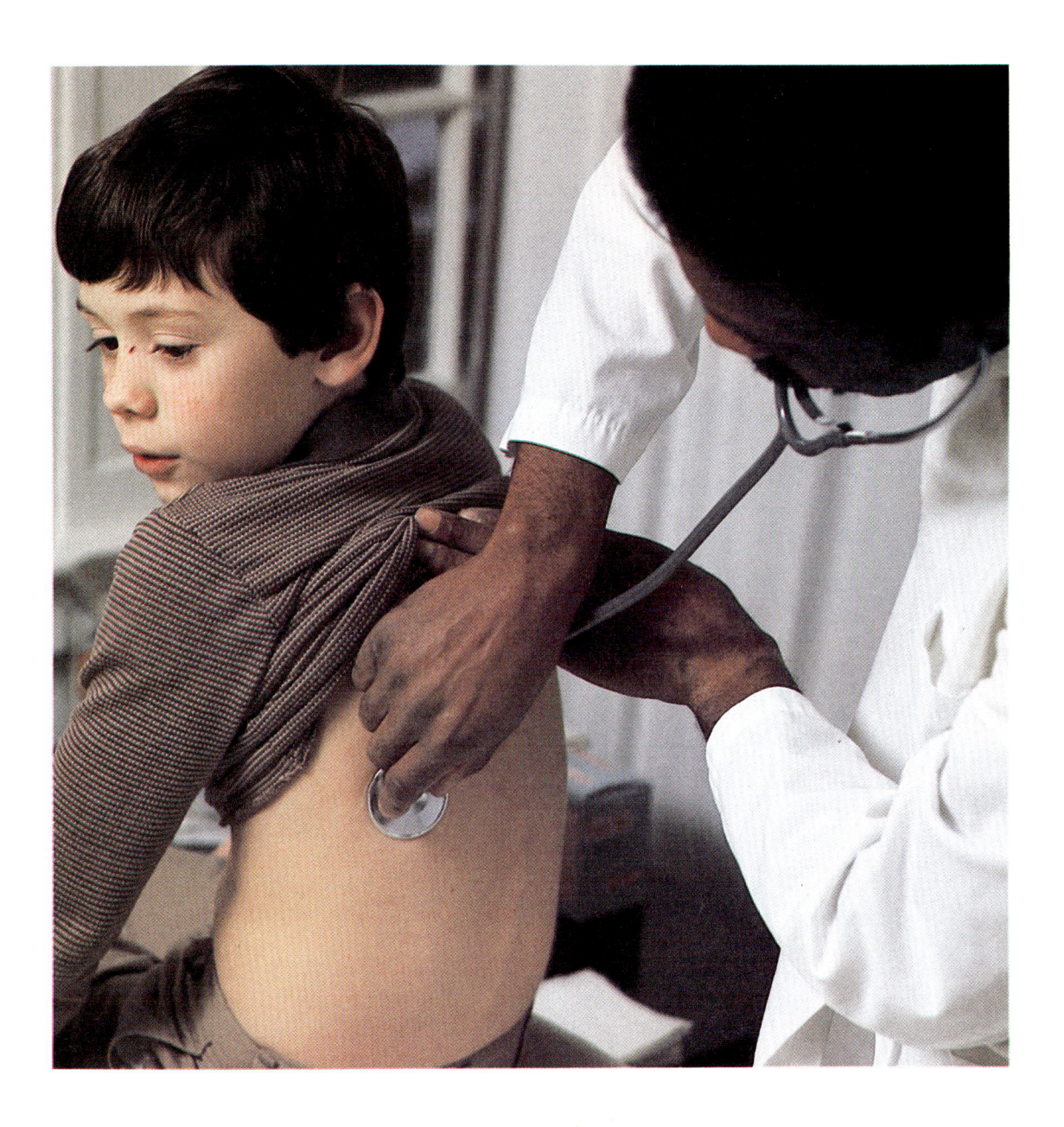

Look at both pictures.

What is the doctor doing?

What else might happen at a check-up?

Why should you get regular check-ups?

Following Good Advice

Sometimes your body may need special care. You might have a cut or a scrape. You might have hurt a muscle or a bone. Doctors and nurses can tell you what to do. Listen to what they say. Follow their advice. Ask a grown-up in your family for help.

Following good advice is important. It can help keep you healthy.

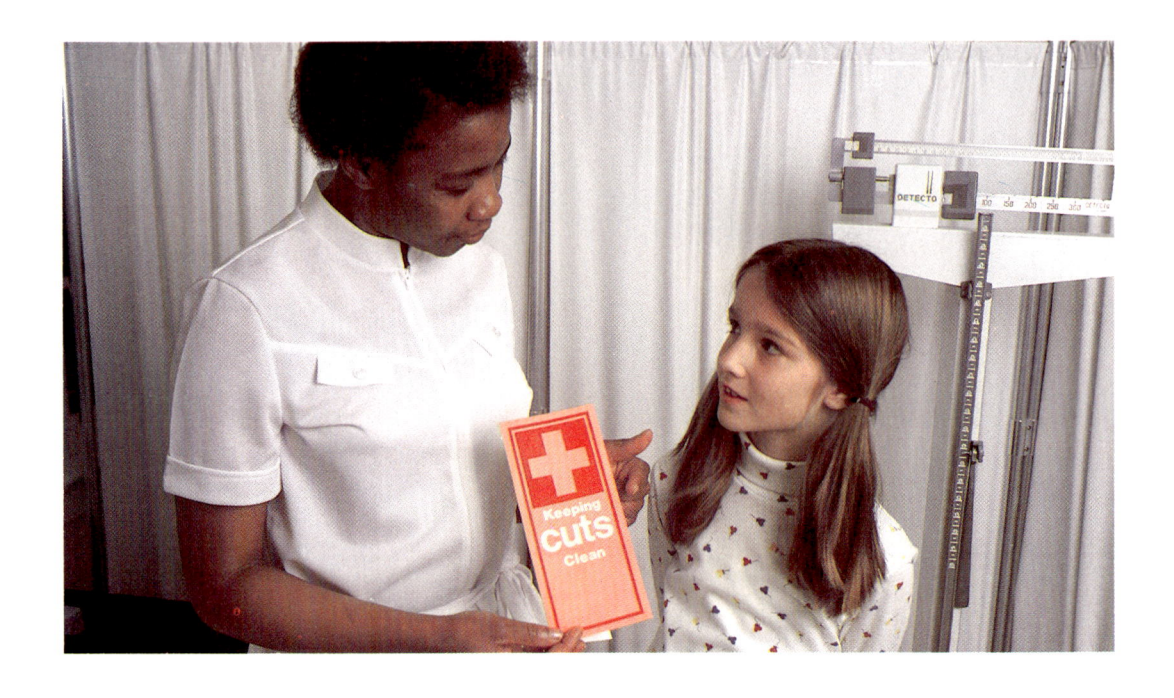

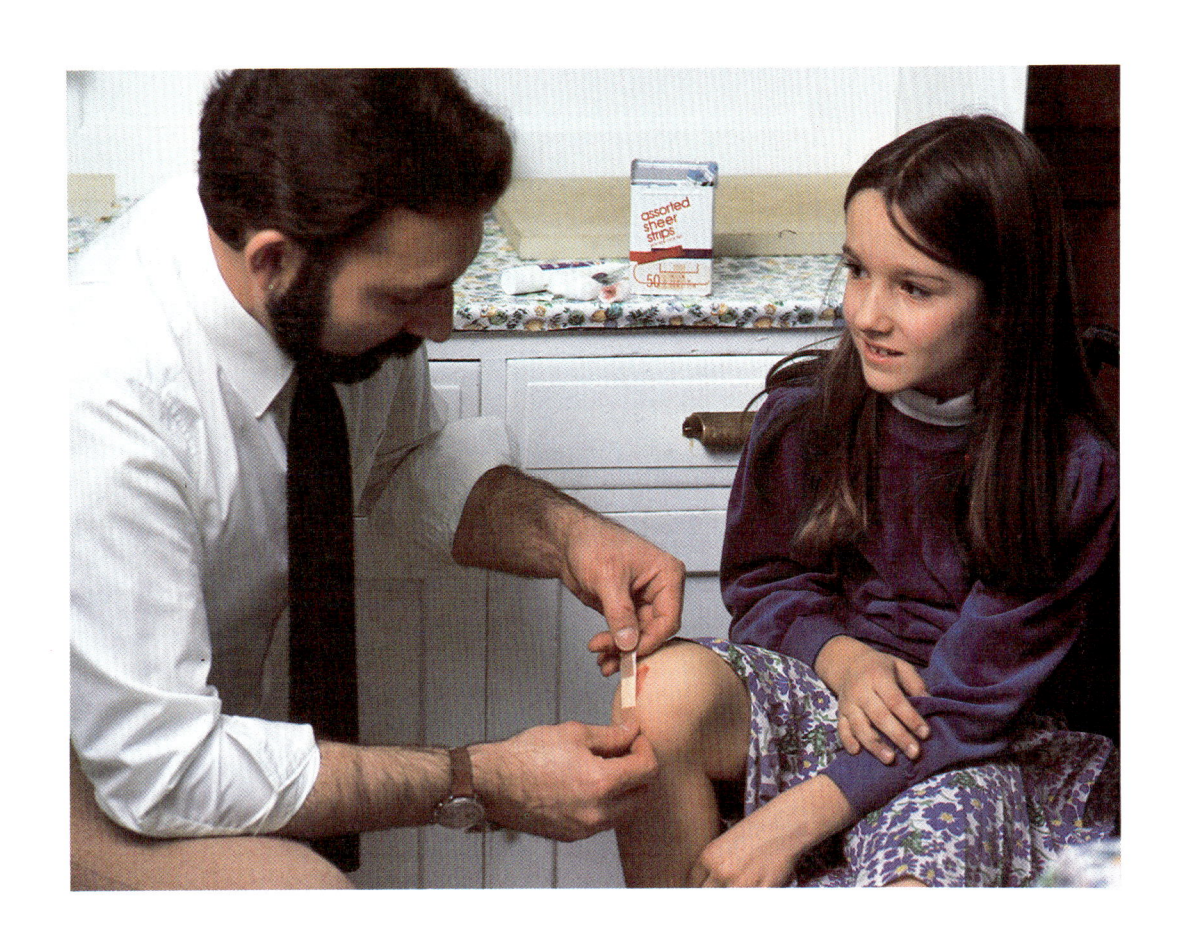

Look at the picture on page 102.
Who is giving good advice?

Look at the picture on this page.
Is the girl following the advice?
How can you tell?
Tell who can give good advice.
Tell why it is important to follow good advice.

Your Turn

Fuzzy Words

David has a new book. It is all about elephants. David likes elephants. He wants to read the book, but he has a problem. The words seem fuzzy.

Tell what David should do.
Tell why your ideas would help.

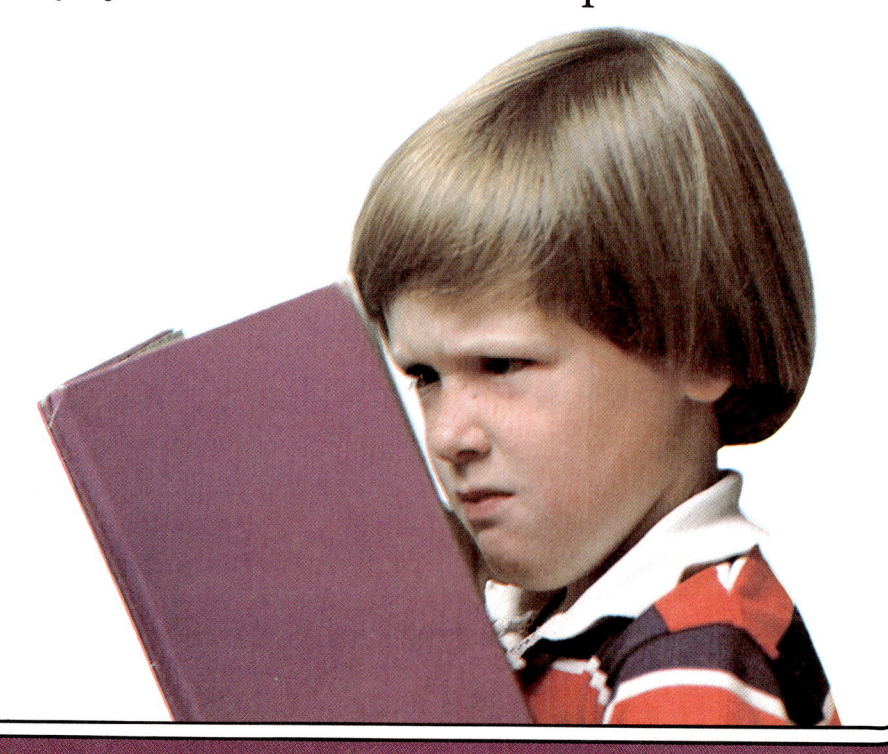

Health in Action

1. Look at the picture. Tell where germs can be found.

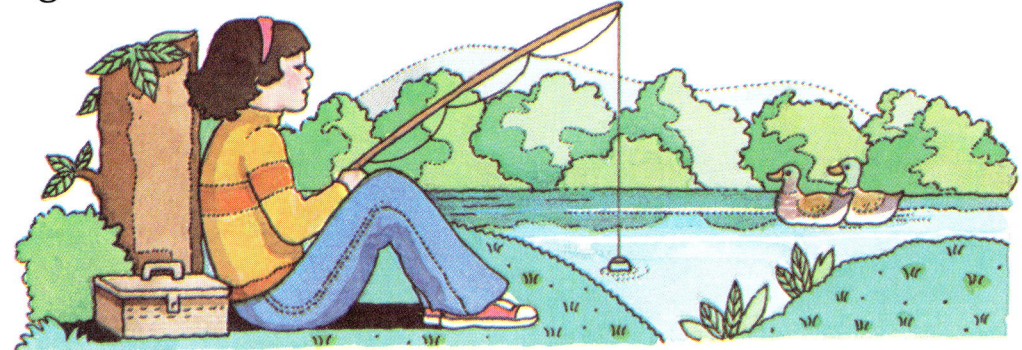

2. Look at the picture again. Pretend everything looks fuzzy. Would you need glasses? Would you want them? Tell why.

3. Name some parts of the body that a doctor checks. Write the names.

4. Write about germs. Tell how they can spread. Tell how you can help keep them from spreading.

Do You Remember?

Your Health Words

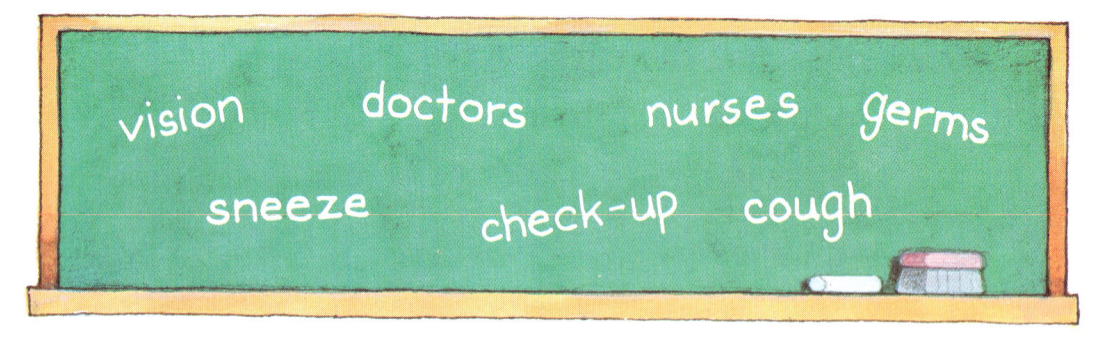

vision   doctors   nurses   germs
sneeze   check-up   cough

Finish the sentences.

Use the Health Words.

1. You can stay well with help from ____.
2. Cover your mouth when you ____.
3. Fuzzy ____ may mean you need glasses.

Your Health Ideas

1. Tell how not to spread germs.
2. Tell what to do if you do not feel well.
3. Tell why you should follow good health advice.

Health Check-Up

Tell which sentences are true.

1. Germs are alive.
2. Germs always stay in one place.
3. There are germs in your mouth.
4. You should go to school with a cold.
5. You should not tell a grown-up when you feel ill.
6. You should keep used tissues.
7. You should let people drink from your cup.
8. It is good to drink juice and water when you have a cold.
9. Doctors can help you learn about your body.
10. You should follow your doctor's advice.

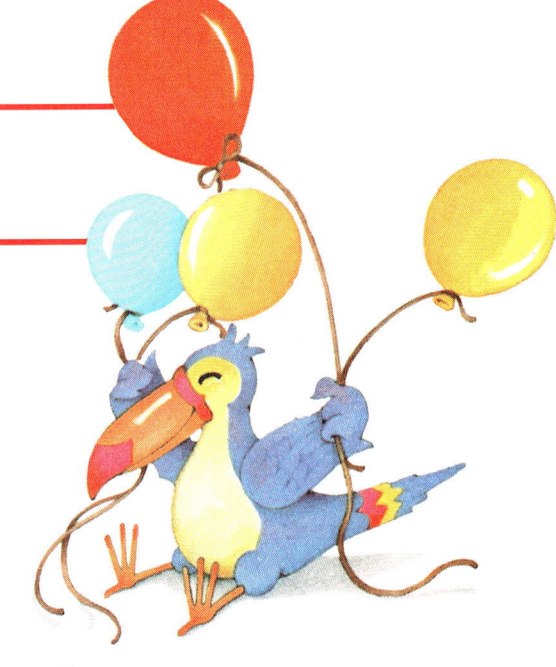

CHAPTER 6

Knowing About Drugs

Almost everything that goes into your body can make a change in it. Food can. Other things can. Some things can help your body. Some are harmful. Learn how each can help or harm you. Be sure the things you take into your body can help.

How can you be sure the things you take into your body can help?

Health Words

medicine   pharmacist
disease   nicotine
drug   tar
poison   caffeine

109

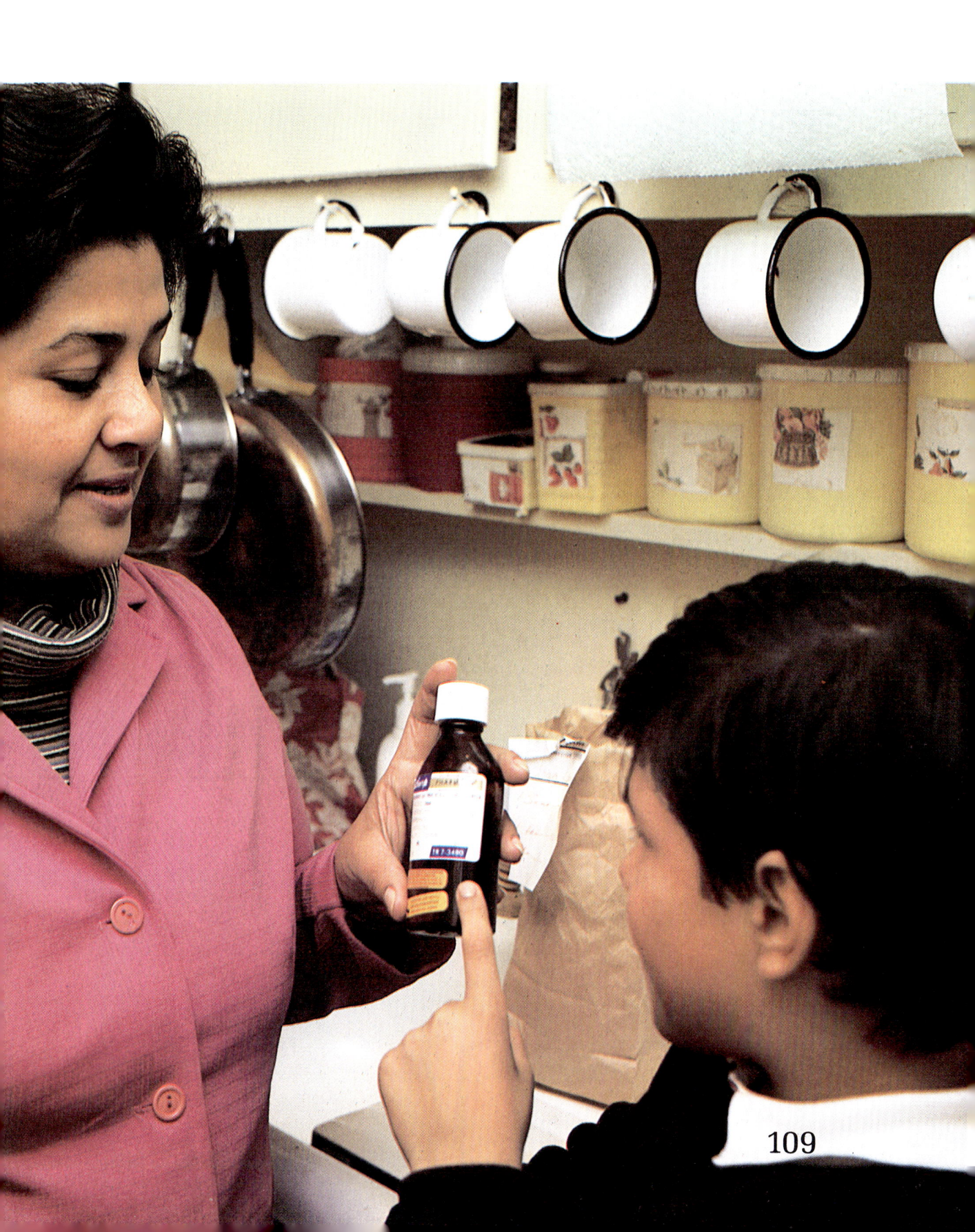

Sometimes Medicine Can Help

Medicines are drugs. They can make a change in the body. Some can help protect the body from disease. Others can help fight germs. Some can fight germs inside the body. Others fight germs on the skin.

Medicines cannot fight all germs, though. They cannot always help.

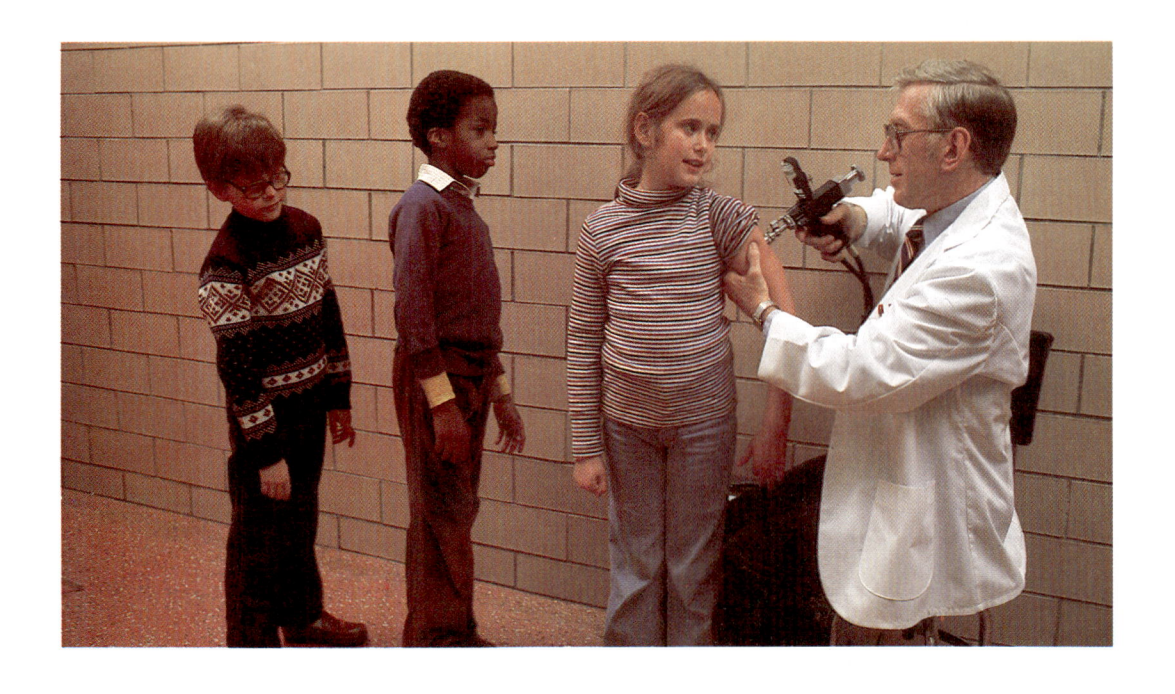

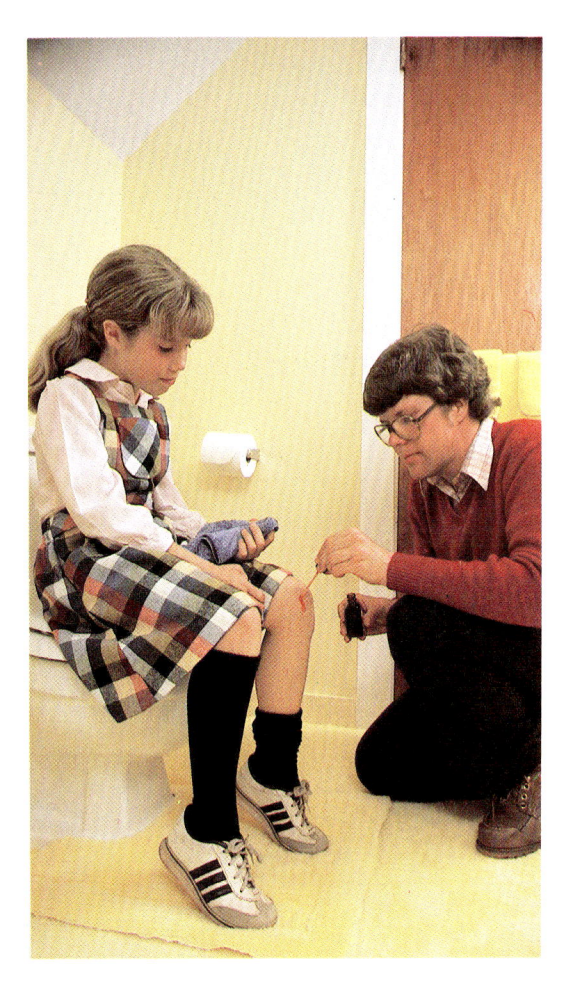

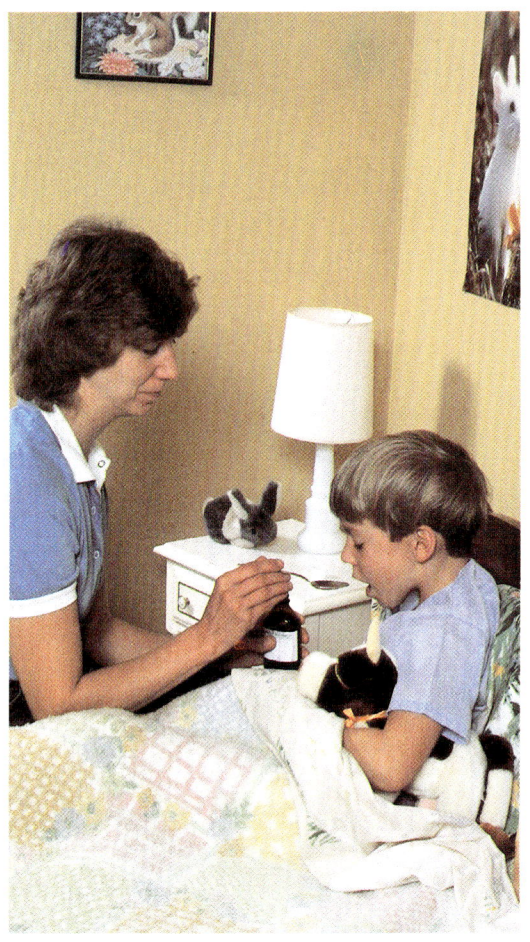

Look at all three pictures.

Which children are getting medicine that can protect them from disease?

Who is getting medicine to help fight germs on the skin?

Can medicine always help?

Tell why or why not.

First, Read the Label

Medicine can help if you use it the way it is supposed to be used. You can find out how to use the medicine you may need. Read the label. Ask a grown-up for help.

Be sure you use medicine in the right way. Always have a grown-up give you the medicine. Always read the label. Always follow directions.

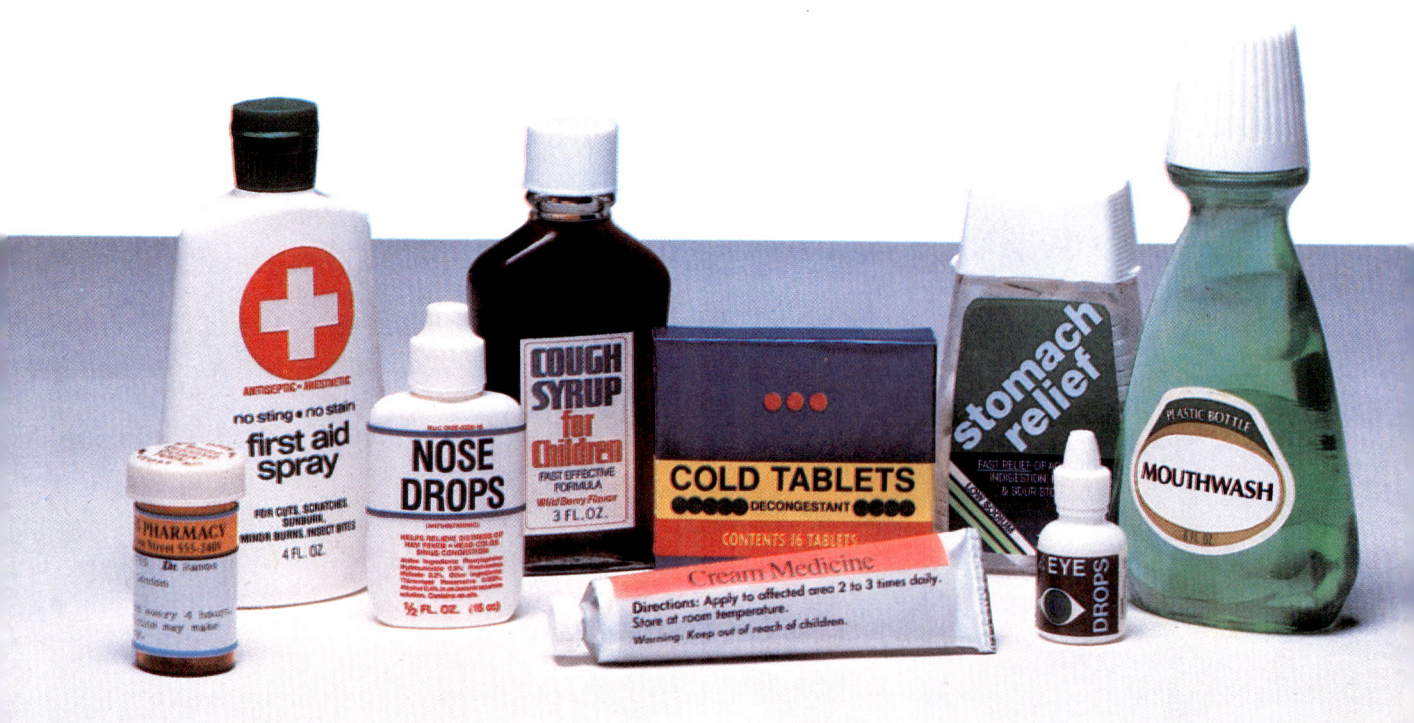

Cough Syrup

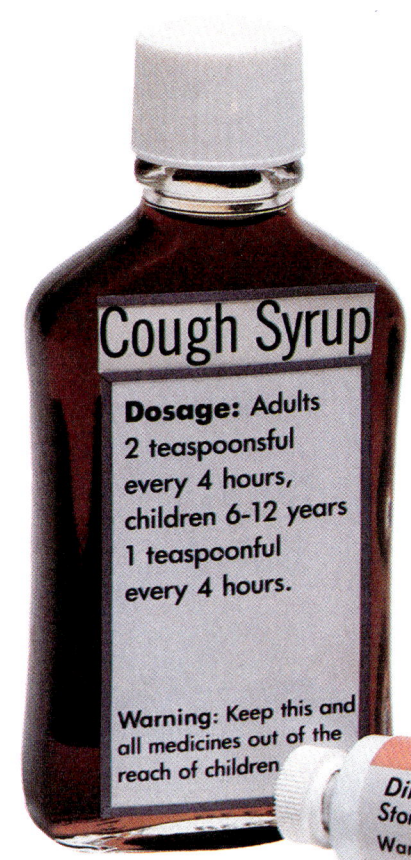

Dosage: Adults 2 teaspoonsful every 4 hours, children 6-12 years 1 teaspoonful every 4 hours.

Warning: Keep this and all medicines out of the reach of children.

Cream Medicine

Directions: Apply to affected area 2 to 3 times daily. Store at room temperature.
Warning: Keep out of reach of children.

Look at the medicines.

Read the labels.

Tell about the medicines.

What kinds of things can you learn about a medicine from reading the label?

Why is it important to read the label?

Why is it important to follow the directions on the label?

Health Highlight

Medicine from Nature

Medicines are drugs. Some drugs are made. Other drugs are not made. They are found in nature. A plant called periwinkle has a drug that can help the bones. A plant called foxglove has a drug that can help the heart. Scientists are learning about other drugs found in plants.

What do some plants have in them?

How can some plants help people?

foxglove

periwinkle

Going, Seeing, and Doing

1. Read the words. Each is the name of a disease. Certain medicines can protect you from these diseases. Copy the words onto your own paper. Find out if you are protected. Ask a grown-up in your family.

   tetanus
   mumps
   measles
   polio

2. Read the label.
   Tell how to use the medicine.

3. Tell what medicine can do.
   Tell what medicine cannot do.

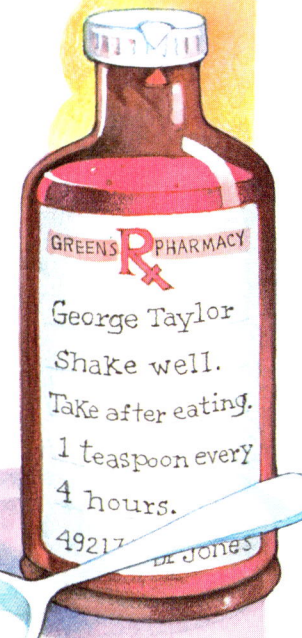

Your Own Medicine

People are different. A medicine that can help one person may not be good for someone else.

Be careful about medicine. Use only your own. Use it only if a grown-up gives it to you. The grown-up could be a doctor or a nurse. It could be a grown-up who is taking care of you. It should be someone who knows about your health.

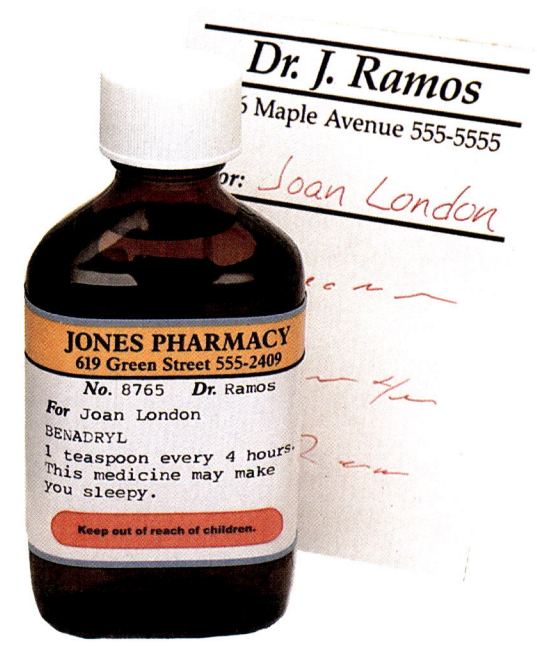

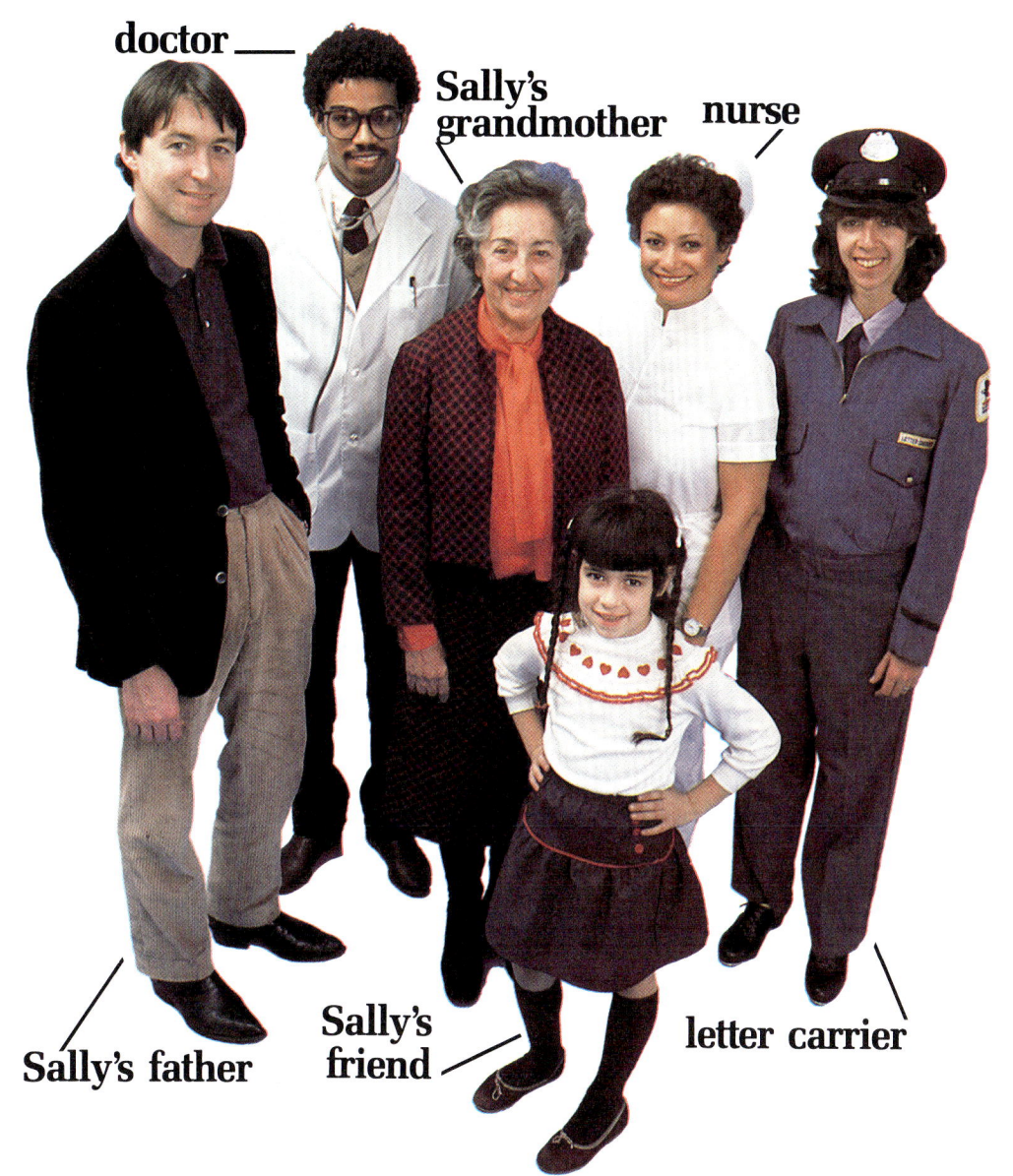

doctor
Sally's grandmother
nurse
Sally's father
Sally's friend
letter carrier

Look at the picture on page 116.
Tell who can use this medicine.
Should you use it?
Tell why.

Look at the picture on this page.
Who can help Sally take medicine safely?

Poisons

Everything you eat and drink goes into your body. Some things can help your body. A poison cannot. A poison can make you very, very ill. Medicine used the wrong way can be a poison.

Some poisons may look like food. Some medicines may, too. Ask a grown-up for help. Ask before you taste.

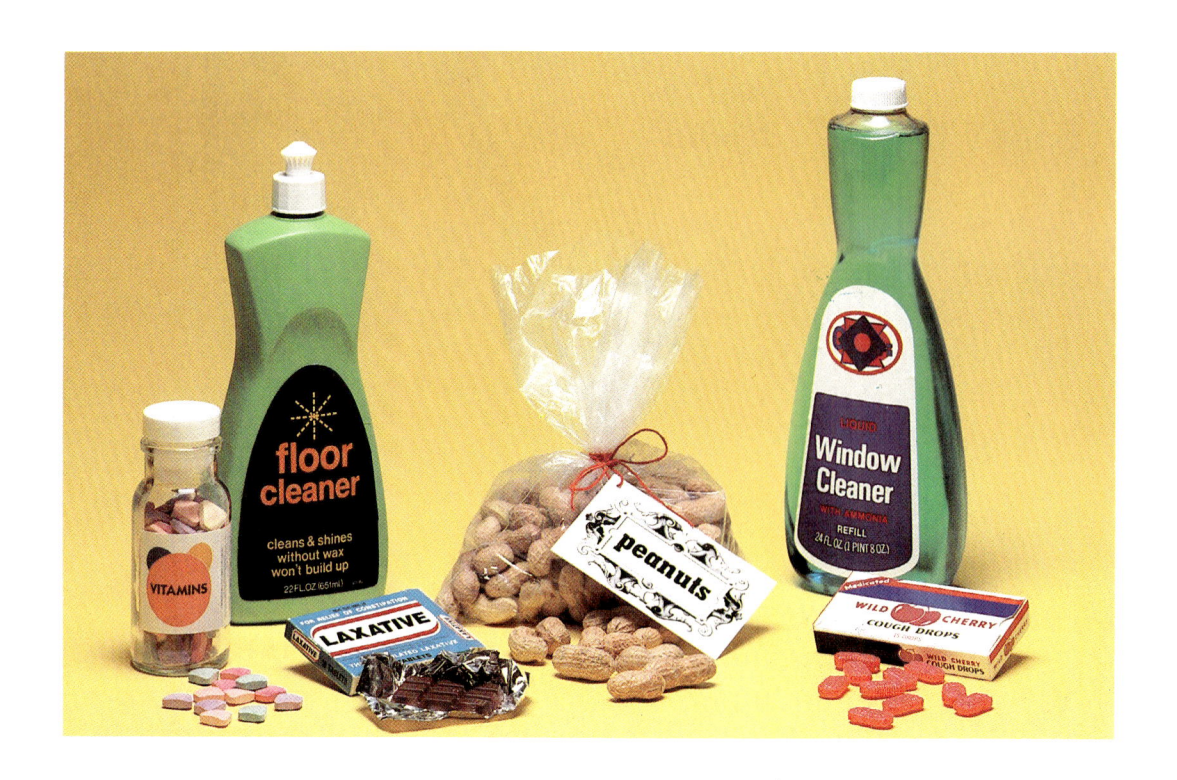

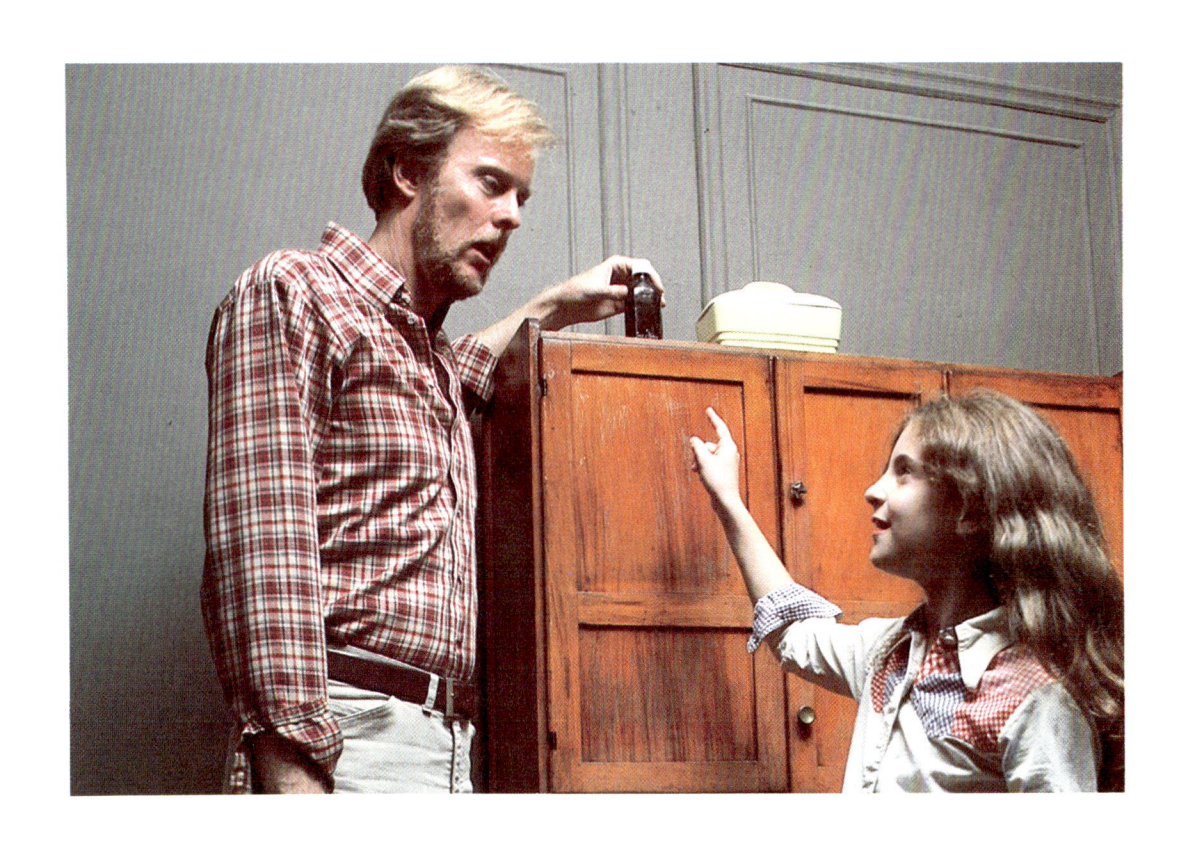

Look at the picture on page 118.

Which are foods?

Which are medicines?

Which are poisons?

Which could be poisons?

Look at the picture on this page.
What is the girl doing?
Why is it important to ask before you taste?

Asking for Help

Learn more about medicines. Ask questions. Ask a doctor or a nurse. Ask a teacher or a grown-up in your family.

Pharmacists can help you, too. Pharmacists are people who may have the medicine you may need. They can tell how the medicine can be used.

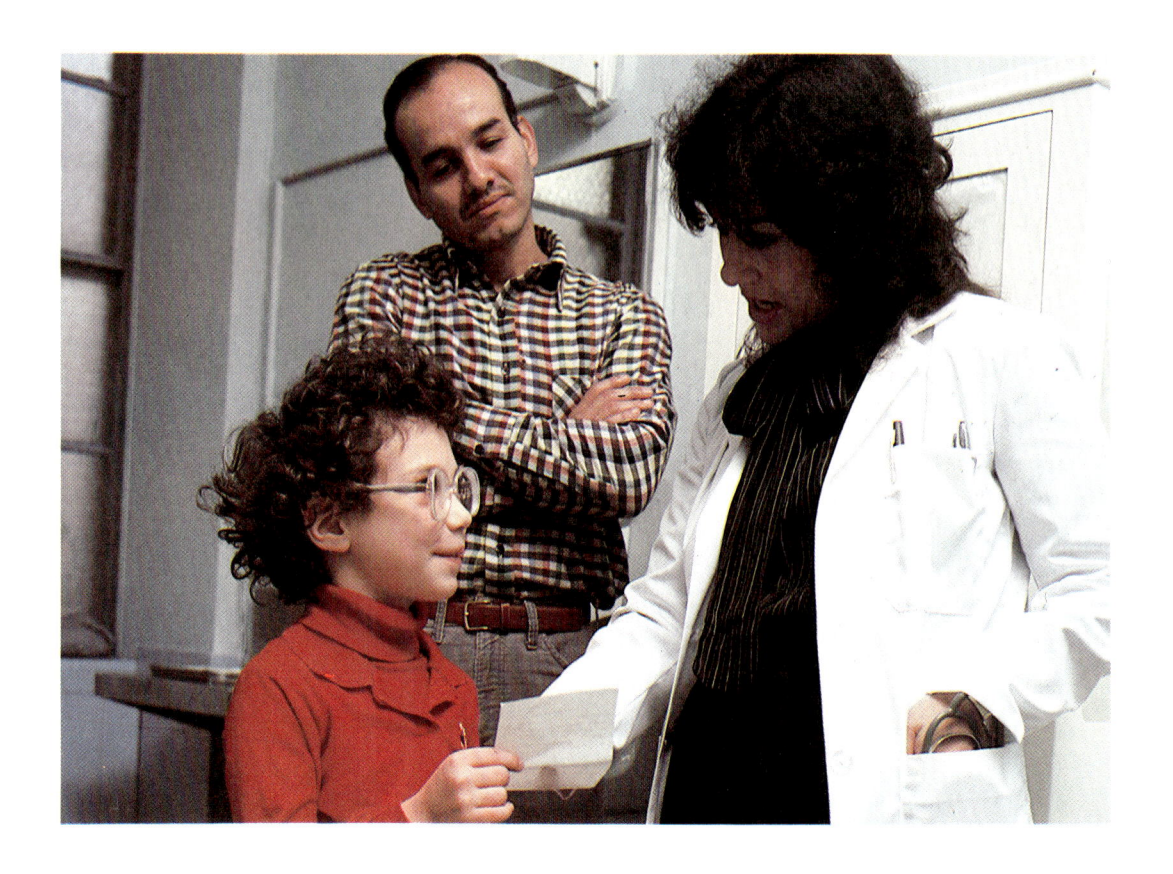

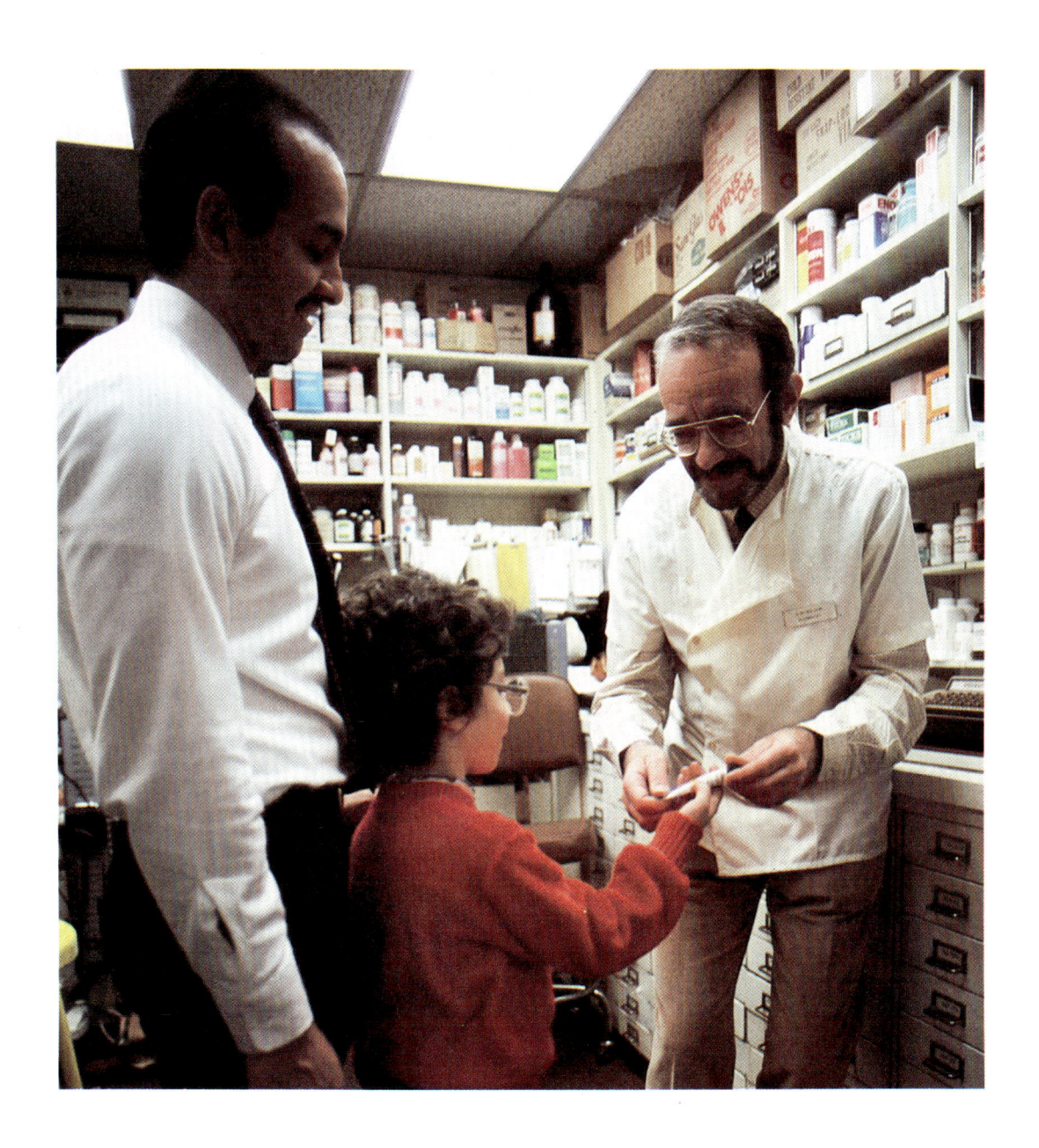

Look at both pictures.

Who is helping the girl learn about medicine in each picture?

Who else could help her learn?

Smoking Isn't Healthy

It is not healthy to smoke. It is not healthy to be around smoke. Tobacco smoke has many drugs in it. One of them is nicotine. Nicotine is harmful. It makes the heart work very hard. Tobacco smoke also has tar in it. Tar can harm the lungs.

Help keep yourself healthy. Try not to breathe tobacco smoke.

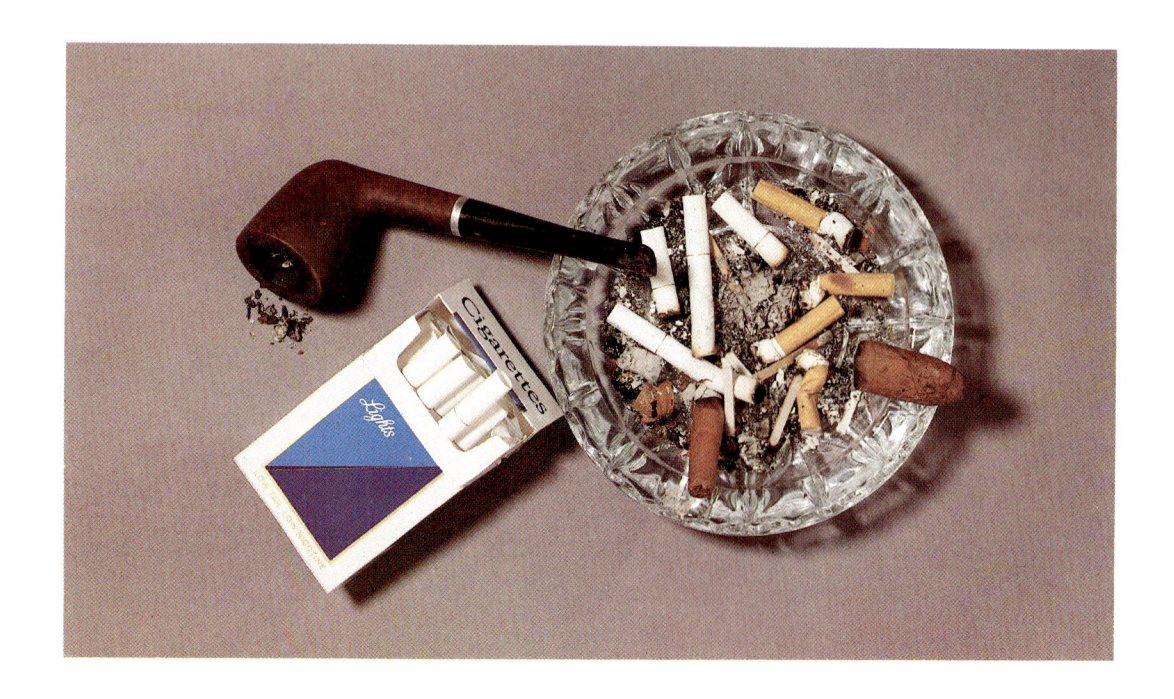

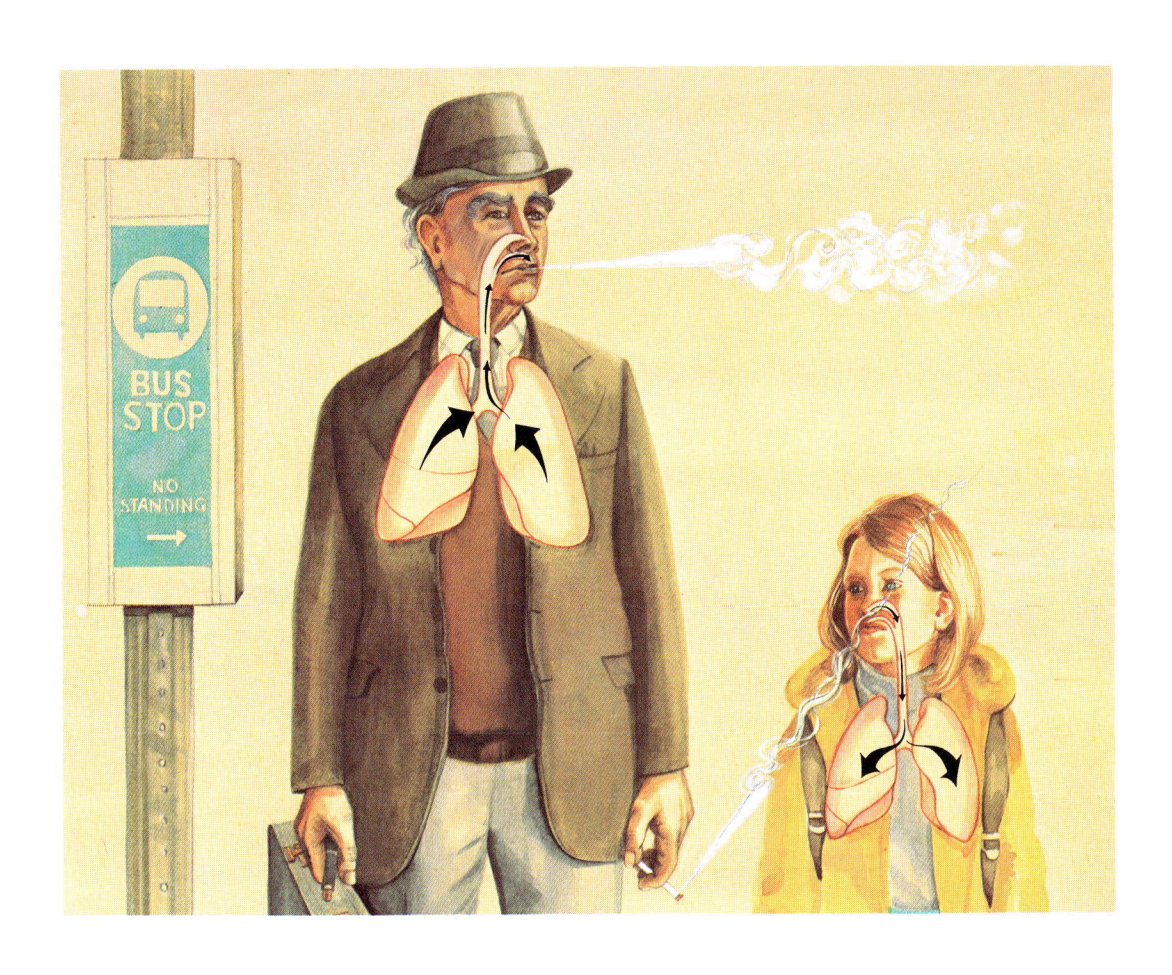

Look at the picture on this page.

Who is being harmed by tobacco smoke?

Where does smoke go when you breathe it?

What can happen to the lungs of people who smoke?

What is one drug in tobacco smoke?

Tell why smoking is not healthy.

Caffeine Isn't Healthy

Caffeine is a drug. It is not good for you. It can make your heart beat faster than it should.

Cola drinks have caffeine. Cocoa does, too. So do foods made from cocoa. These foods are not good for you.

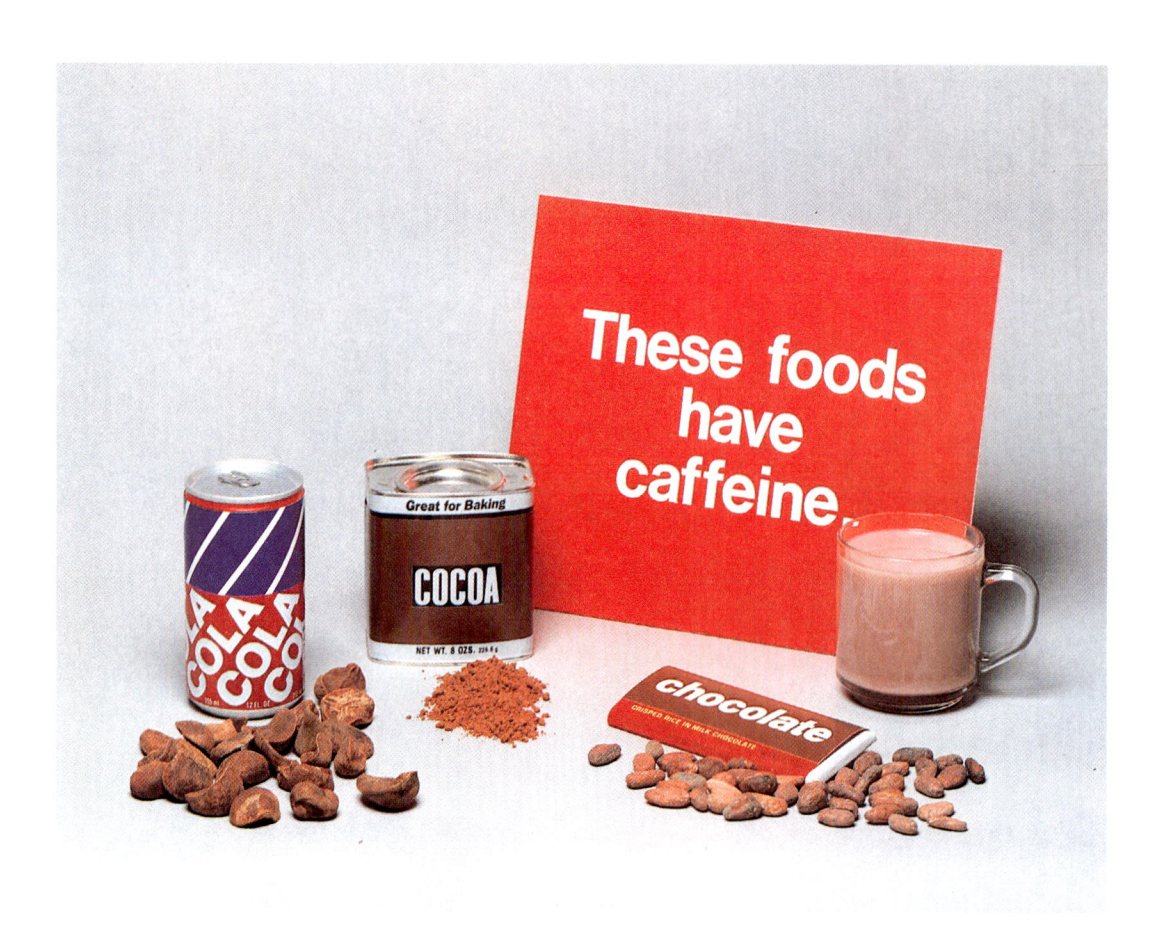

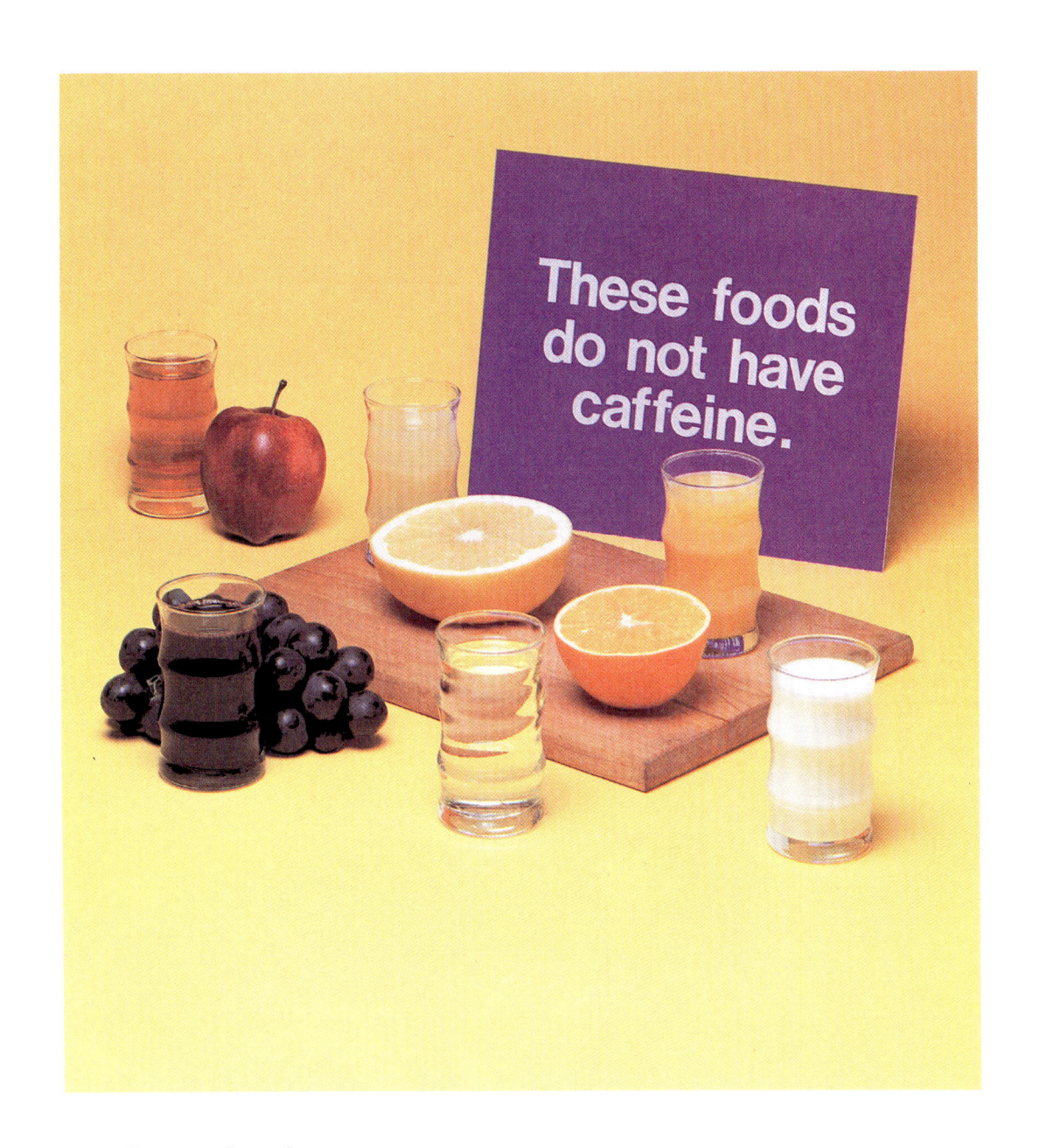

Look at both pictures.

Which foods should you choose?

Tell why.

Tell what caffeine can do to the body.

Your Turn

Making a Healthful Choice

Lucy is thirsty. She wants something to drink. There are many drinks to choose from. She can't decide.

Help Lucy.
Help her choose a healthful drink.
Tell why the drink is healthful.

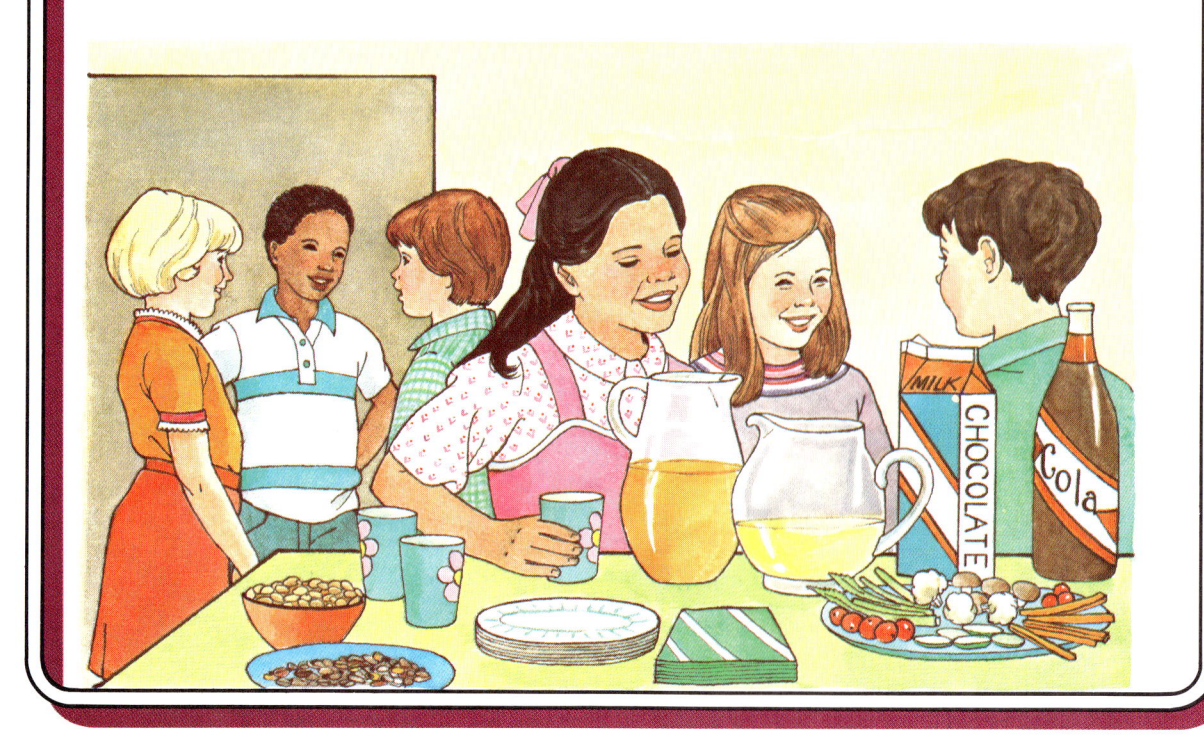

Health in Action

1. Look at the pictures. Tell why you should ask about these things. Tell whom you should ask.

2. Make believe you are in a room. Someone near you is smoking. You want to be polite, but you do not want to breathe in smoke. Tell what you would do.

3. List some rules about medicine. Tell how to use it safely.

4. Write about caffeine. Tell what it is. Tell what caffeine does to the body. Name some foods that have caffeine.

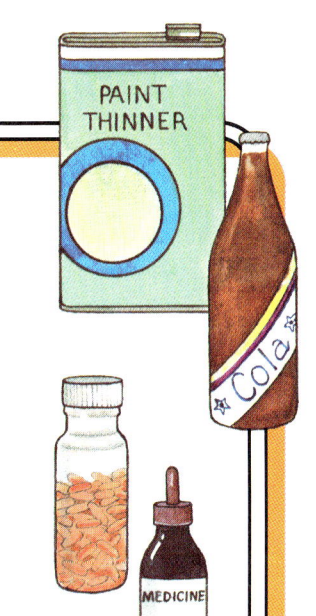

Do You Remember?

Your Health Words

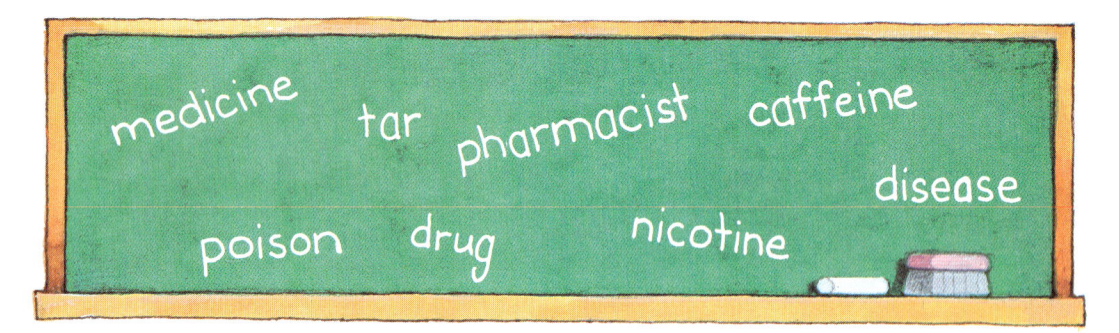

medicine tar pharmacist caffeine disease poison drug nicotine

Answer the questions.
Use the Health Words.

1. Which are drugs?
2. Which drugs are harmful?
3. Who can help you learn about medicine?

Your Health Ideas

1. Tell why medicine labels are important.
2. Tell why smoking isn't healthy.
3. Tell why you should ask about things before you eat or drink them.

Health Check-Up

Tell which sentences are true.

1. All medicine is used inside the body.
2. Some medicine can help protect the body from disease.
3. You should share your medicine.
4. A pharmacist can answer questions about medicine.
5. You should take only your own medicine.
6. Never read a medicine label.
7. Nicotine and caffeine are drugs.
8. Caffeine is good for you.
9. Medicine can always help you.
10. Tobacco smoke is bad for you.

CHAPTER 7

Safety in Your World

Help protect yourself and others from injury. Learn to cross a street safely. Play safely indoors and out. Ride a bicycle safely. Ride in buses and cars safely. Act safely around animals. You are a very important person. Help keep yourself safe. Help keep others safe, too.

How can you help keep yourself and others safe?

Health Words

safety   crossing guard   lifeguard
traffic   seatbelt   first aid
crosswalk   accidents

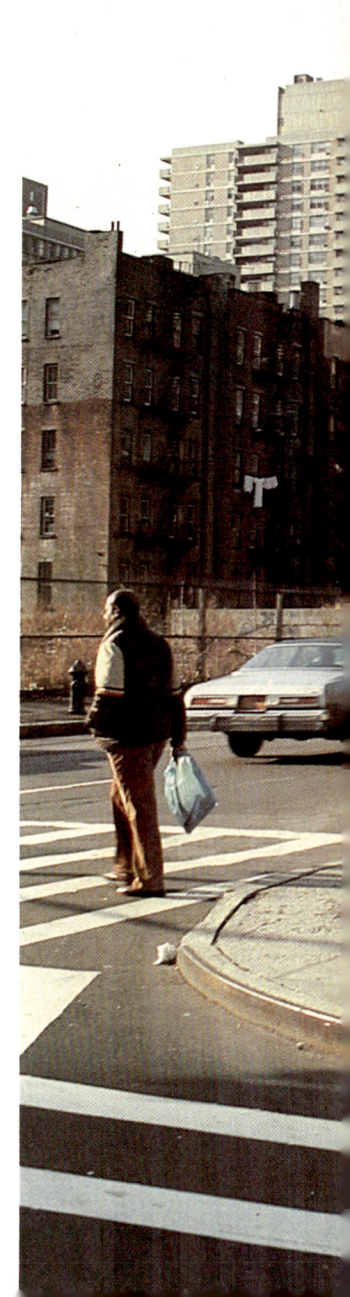

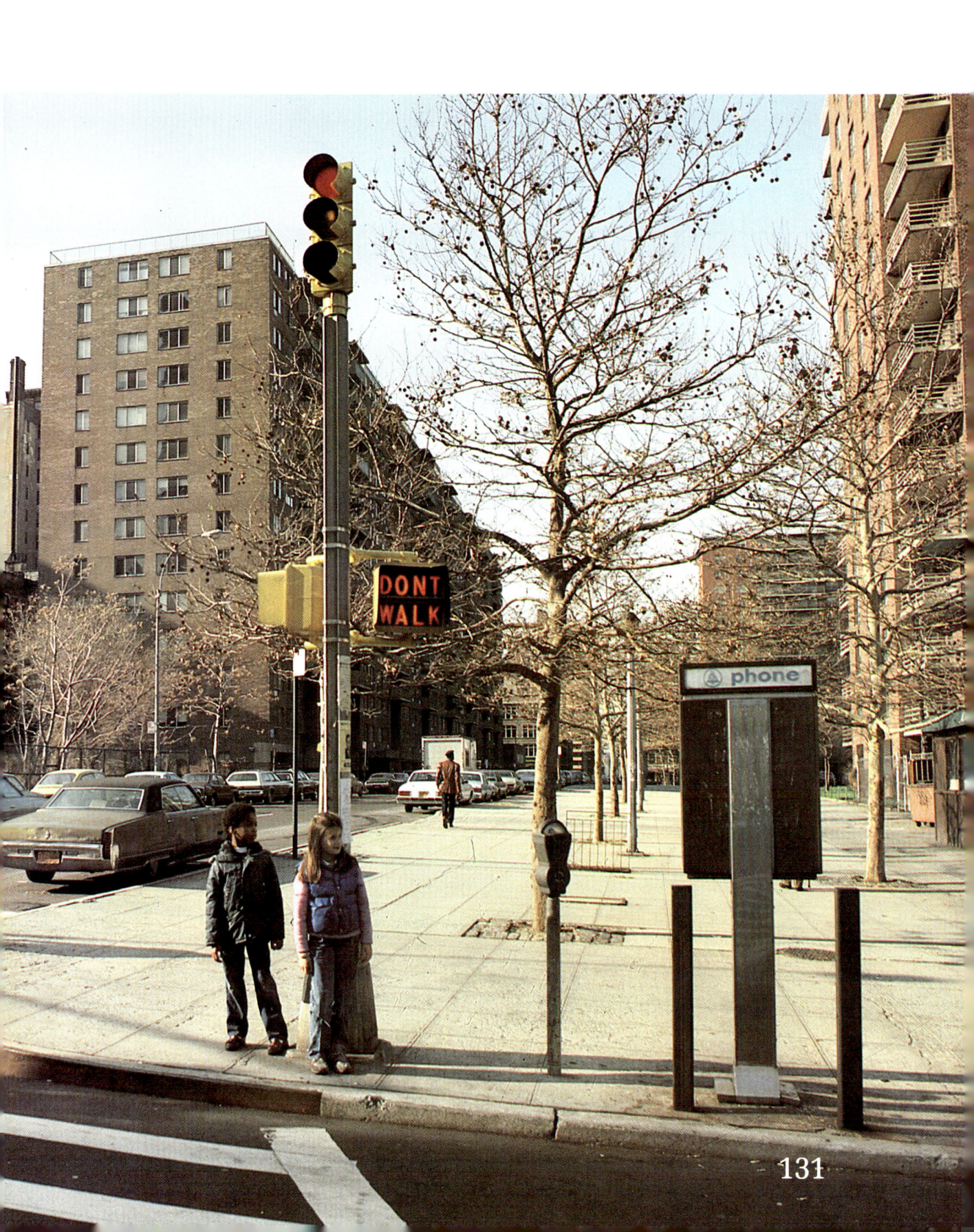

Cars, Corners, and Crosswalks

Streets can be busy with traffic. You can learn to cross safely, though. Follow these safety rules.

Cross only at corners or crosswalks. Obey the traffic light. Obey the crossing guard. Before you cross, look both ways. Be sure traffic has stopped.

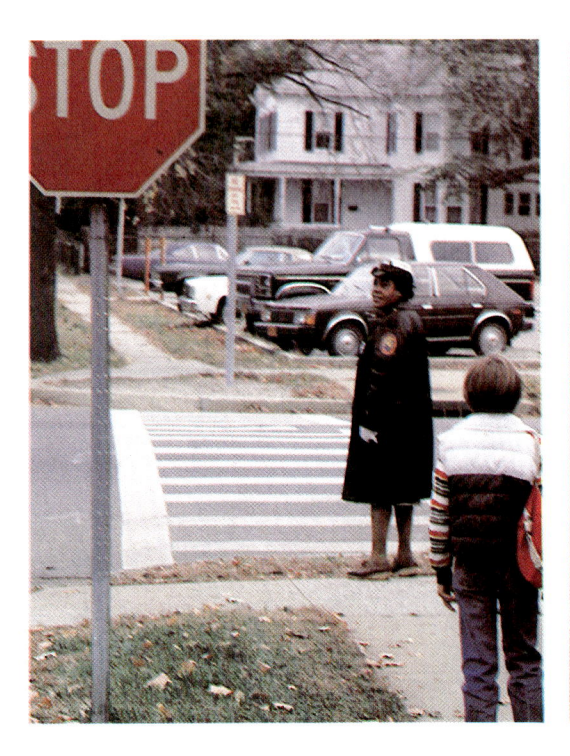

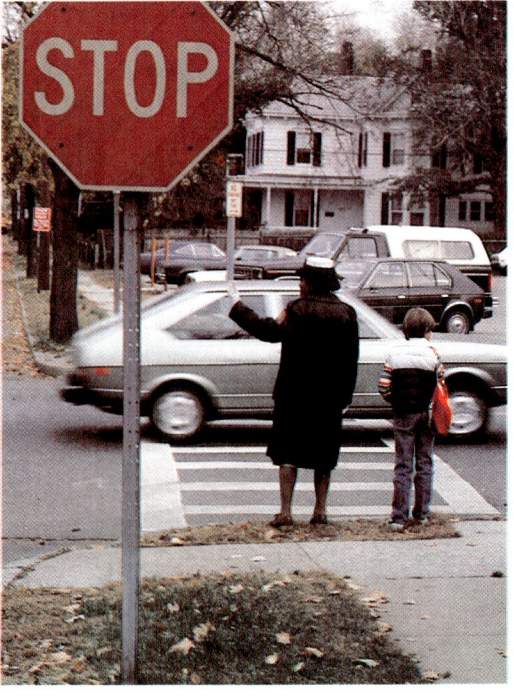

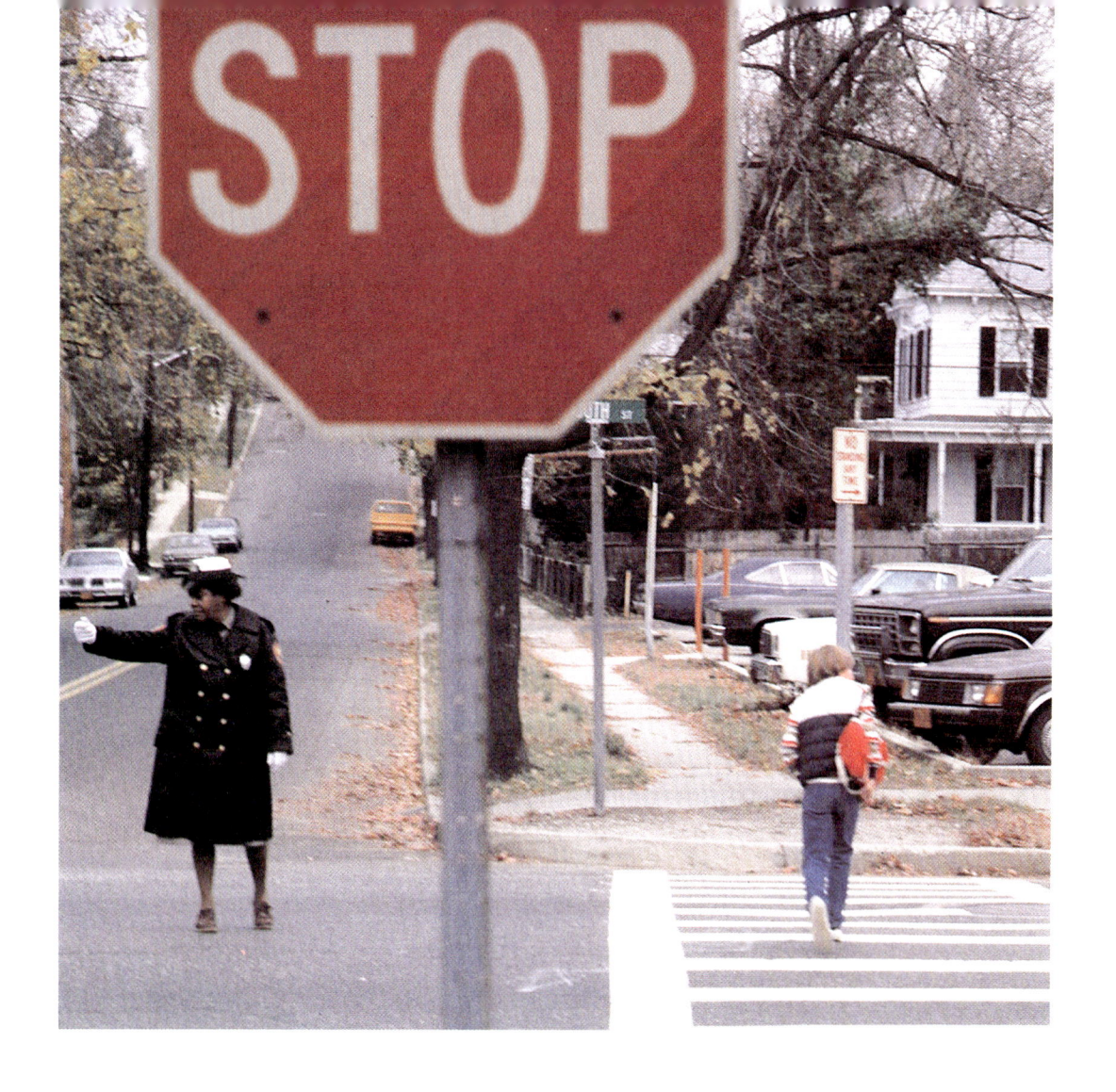

Look at the pictures on page 132.

Who is helping the boy cross the street?

Is it safe to cross?

How do you know?

Look at the picture on this page.

Tell why it is safe to cross.

Tell how to cross a street safely.

Riding Bicycles

You can learn to ride a bicycle safely. Stay to the right. Ride in single file. Ride alone on your bicycle. Watch out for traffic. Follow the safety rules for crossing a street. Never ride into the street from between parked cars.

Learn other bicycle safety rules. Follow them every time you ride.

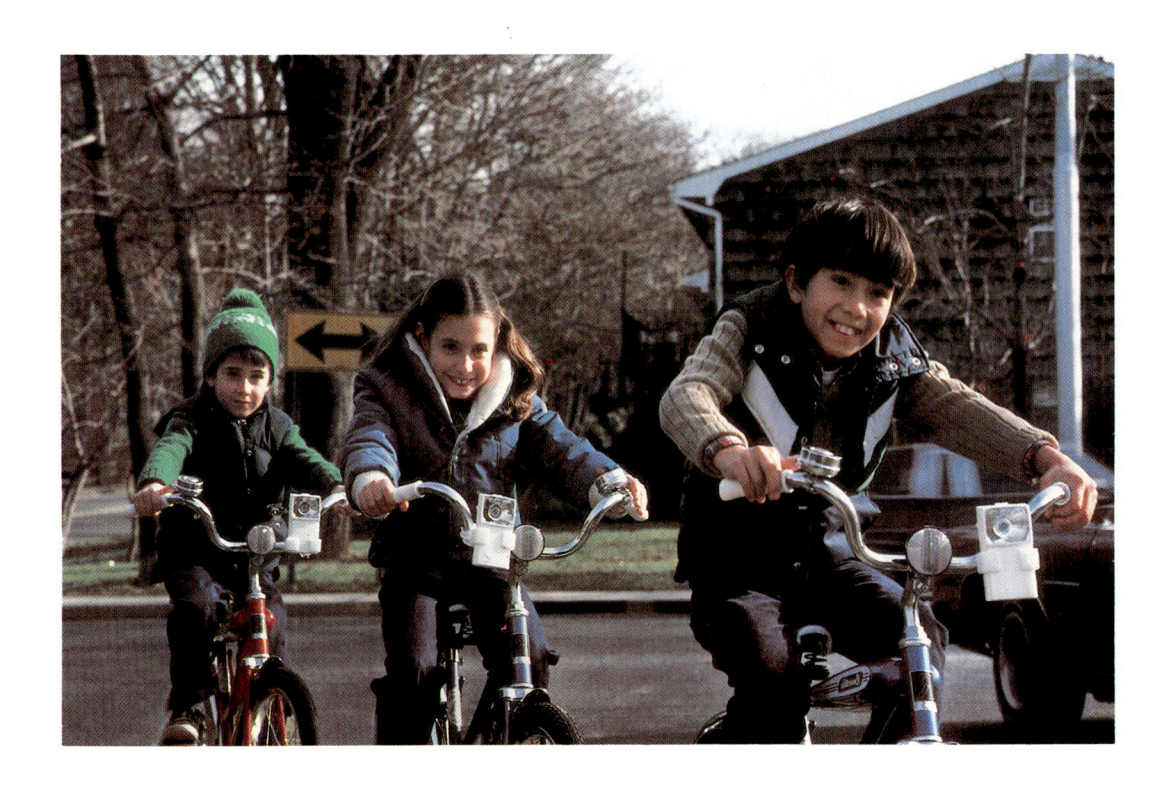

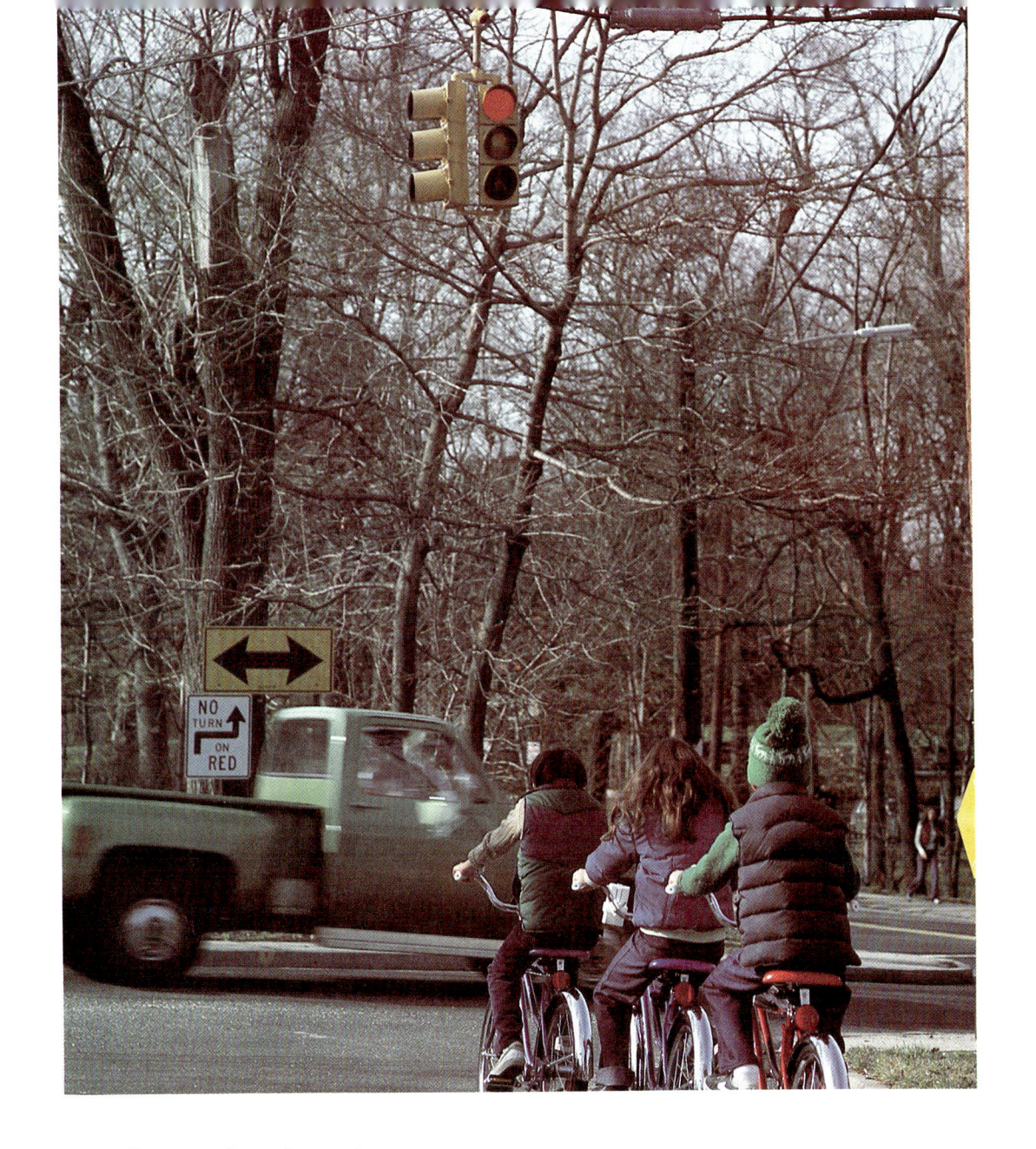

Look at both pictures.

Are the children riding safely?

How can you tell?

Tell about some other bicycle safety rules.

Tell why riding safely is important.

Health Highlight

The First Bicycle Tires

Long ago, bicycles were not safe. They had metal wheels. The bicycles tipped easily.

John Dunlop decided to do something about it. He got some rubber tubes. He filled them with air. Then, he put the tubes on his son's tricycle. They were the very first tires. They helped keep the tricycle from tipping.

How do tires help make bicycles safe? Name some other things that help.

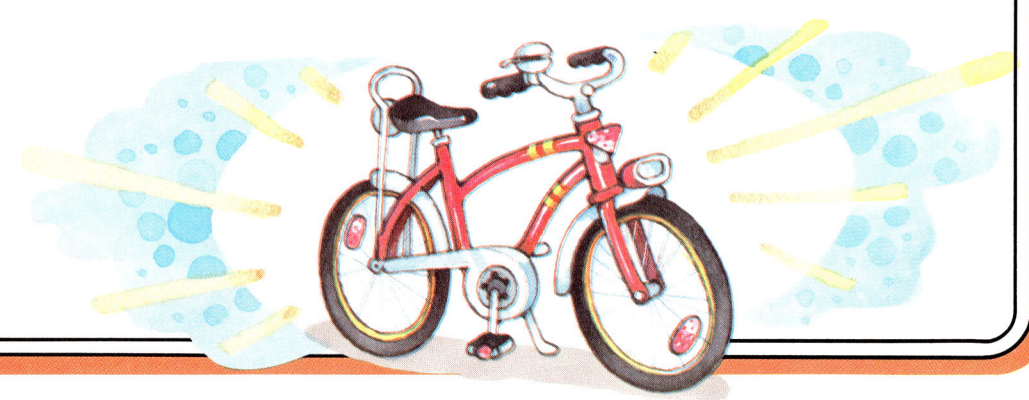

Going, Seeing, and Doing

1. Find out more about safety rules for crossing a street. Ask a crossing guard or a police officer. Follow his or her advice.

2. Stand on a corner near school. Stay there for a few minutes. Watch people as they cross the street. Are they following safety rules? Which rules? How can these rules help keep them safe?

3. Work with your classmates. Make a list of bicycle safety rules. Follow the rules whenever you ride a bicycle.

Riding in Buses and Cars

Ride safely in buses and cars. Use seatbelts whenever you can. Talk quietly. Stay in your seat. Keep your arms and legs inside the windows. Doing these things helps the driver drive safely.

Follow these safety rules whenever you travel. Help keep yourself and others safe for the next trip.

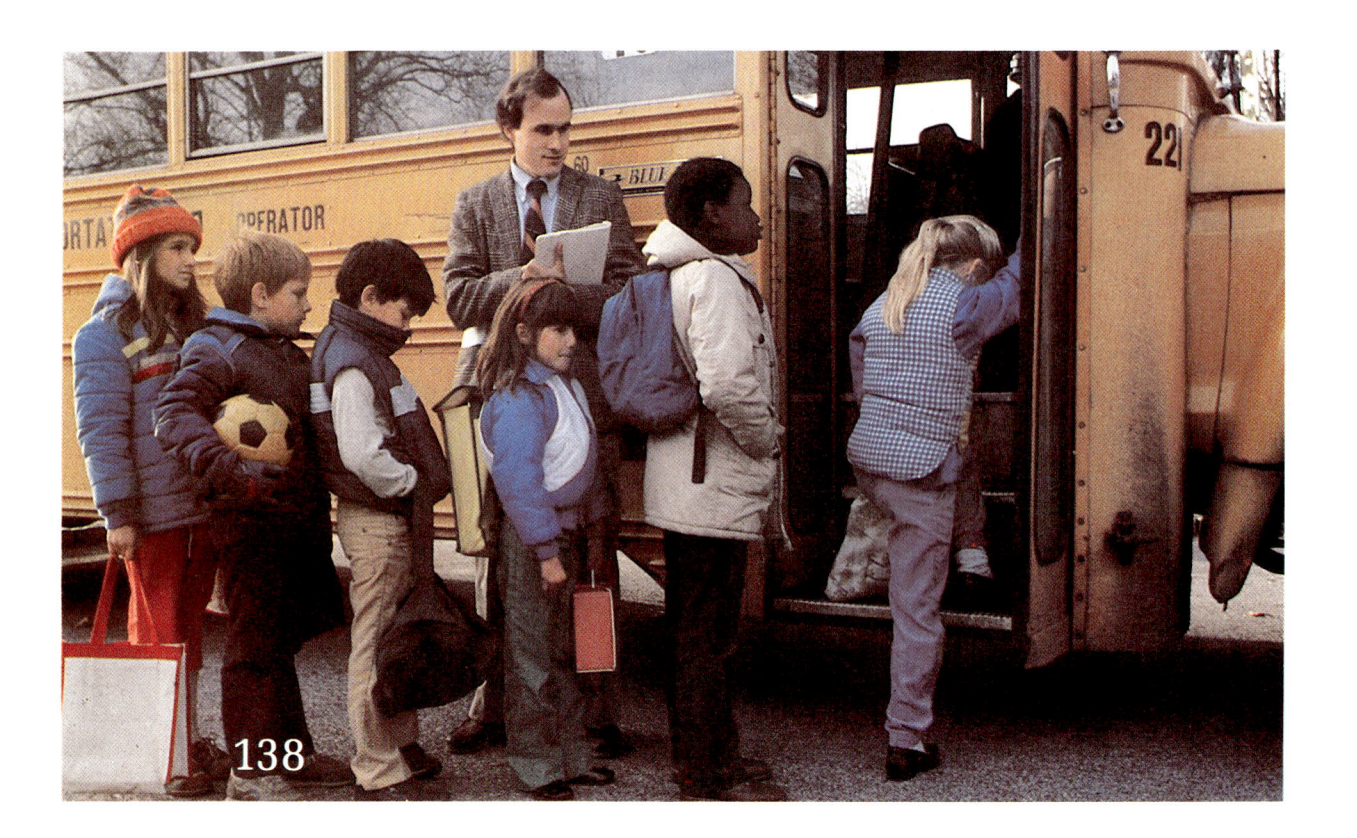

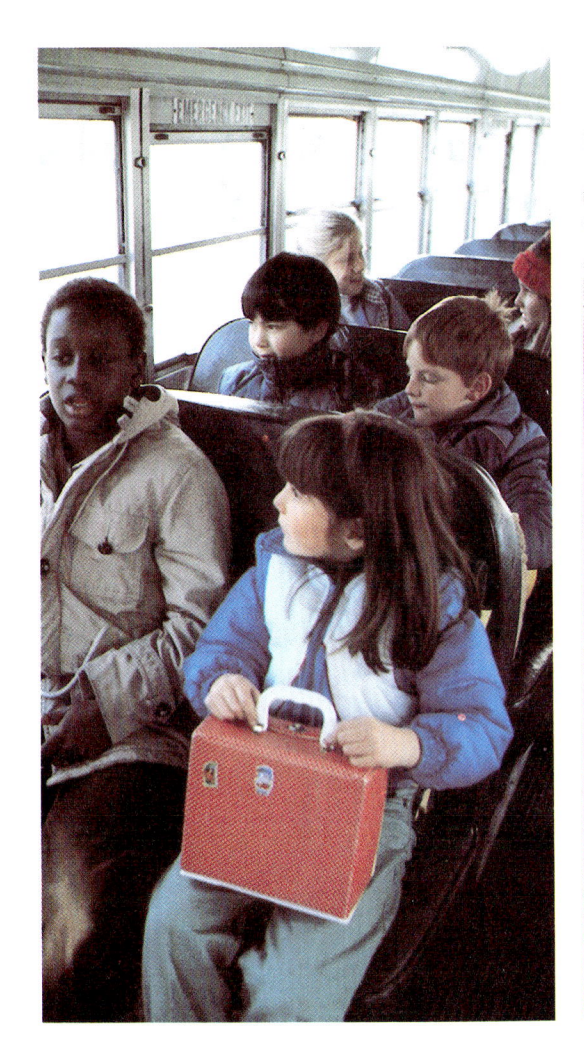

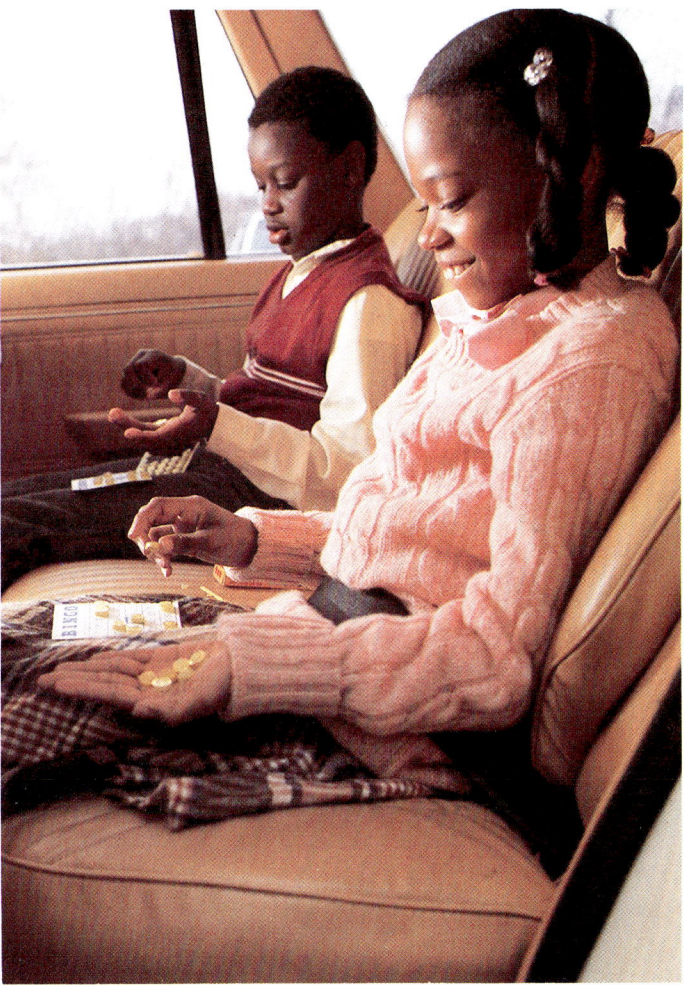

Look at all three pictures.

What safety rules are the children following?

Why are these rules important?

Name some safe games for a car or bus trip.

139

Being Careful Around Animals

Animals can be fun when you treat them safely. Don't make sudden moves around them. Don't make loud noises. Never tease or grab at them. They may try to bite or scratch you.

Be extra careful when the owner is not nearby. Keep your distance. Walk away slowly. Think about your safety.

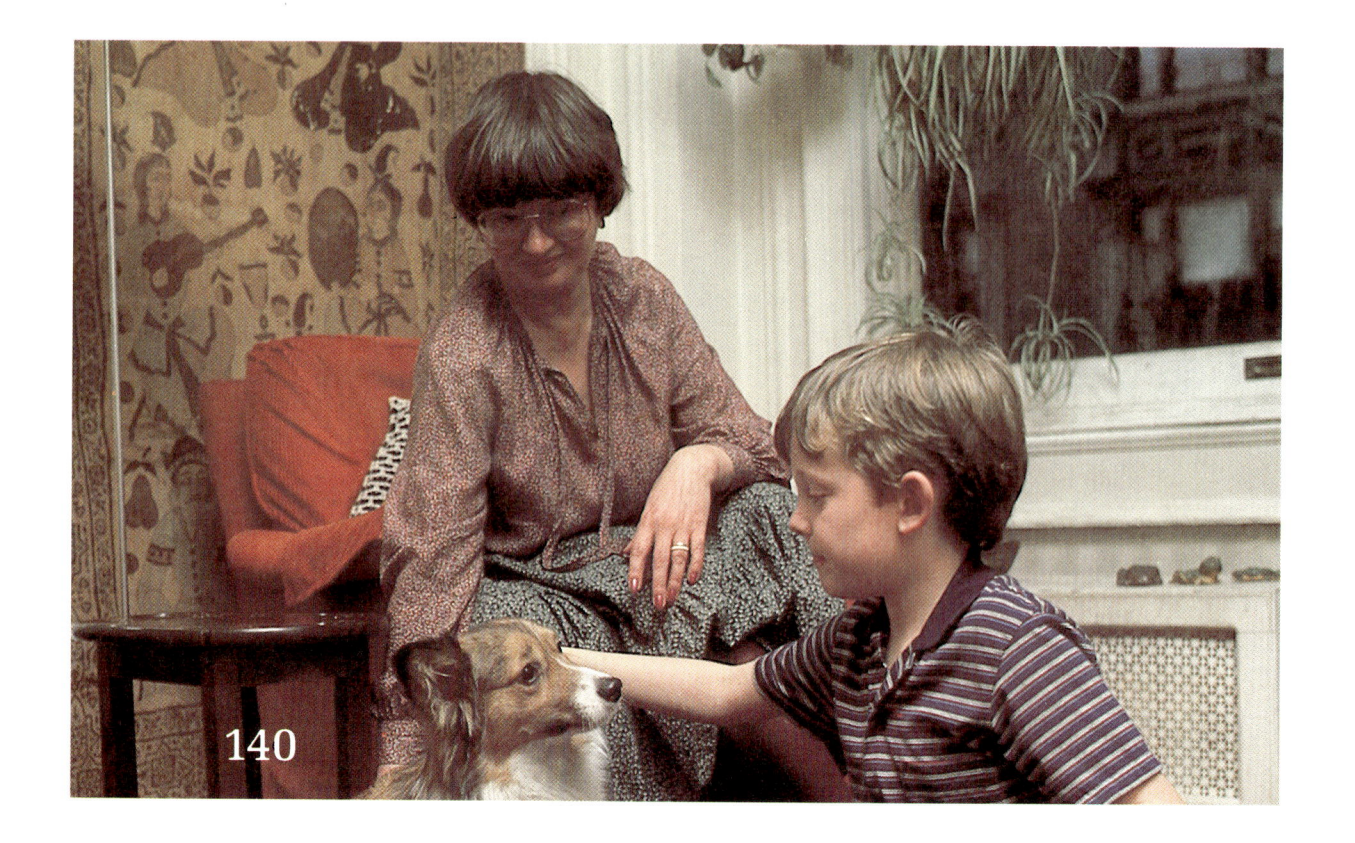

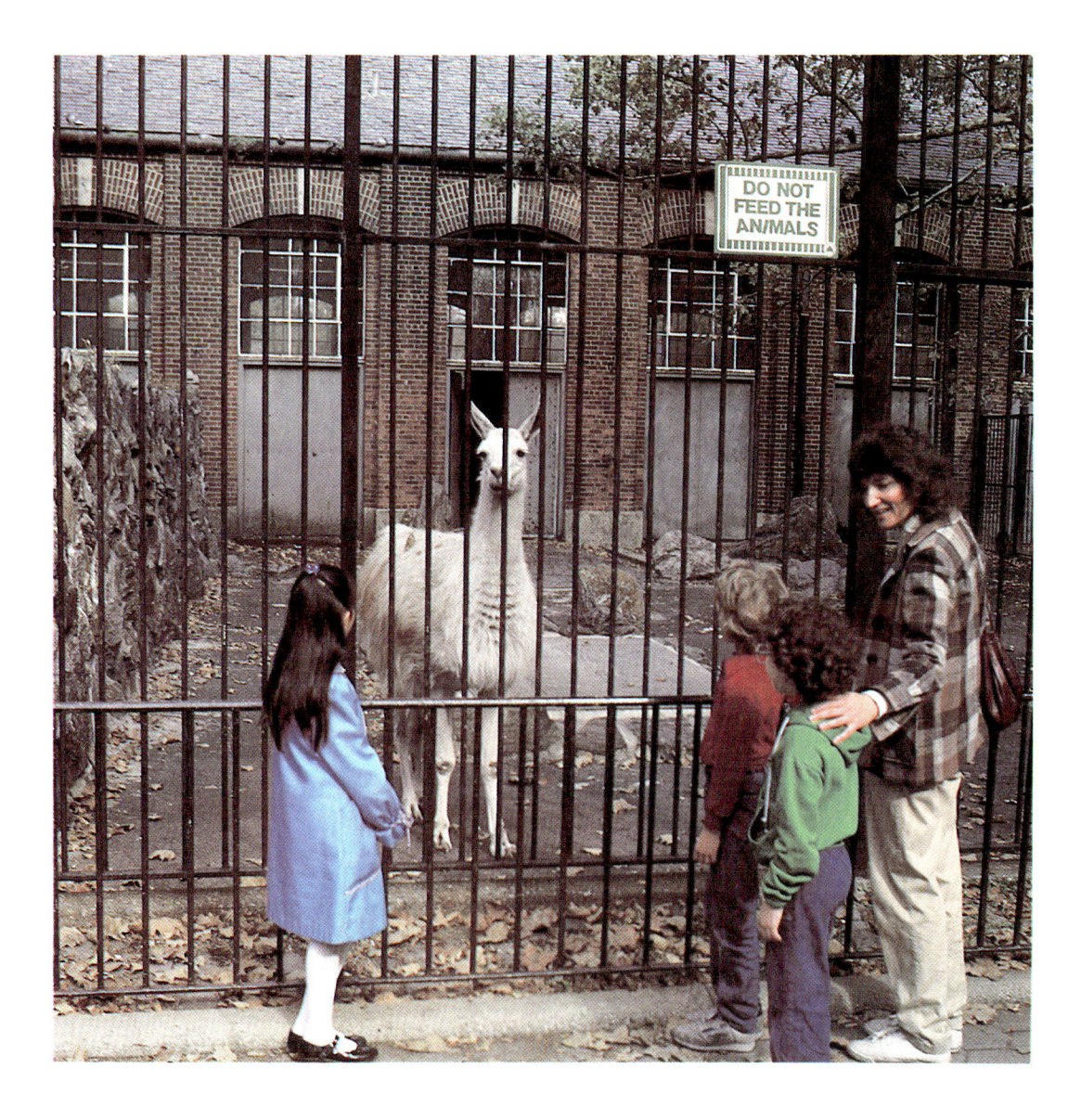

Look at both pictures.

Are the children being safe around animals?

How can you tell?

How else can you be safe around animals?

Tell why safety around animals is important.

141

Safety Outside

Play safely outside. Use slides the way they are meant to be used. Use all play things the way they are meant to be used. Play running games only where there is room to run. Don't play them near slides or swings.

Be safe in the water, too. Swim only when there is a lifeguard to watch you. Swim with a friend or a grown-up.

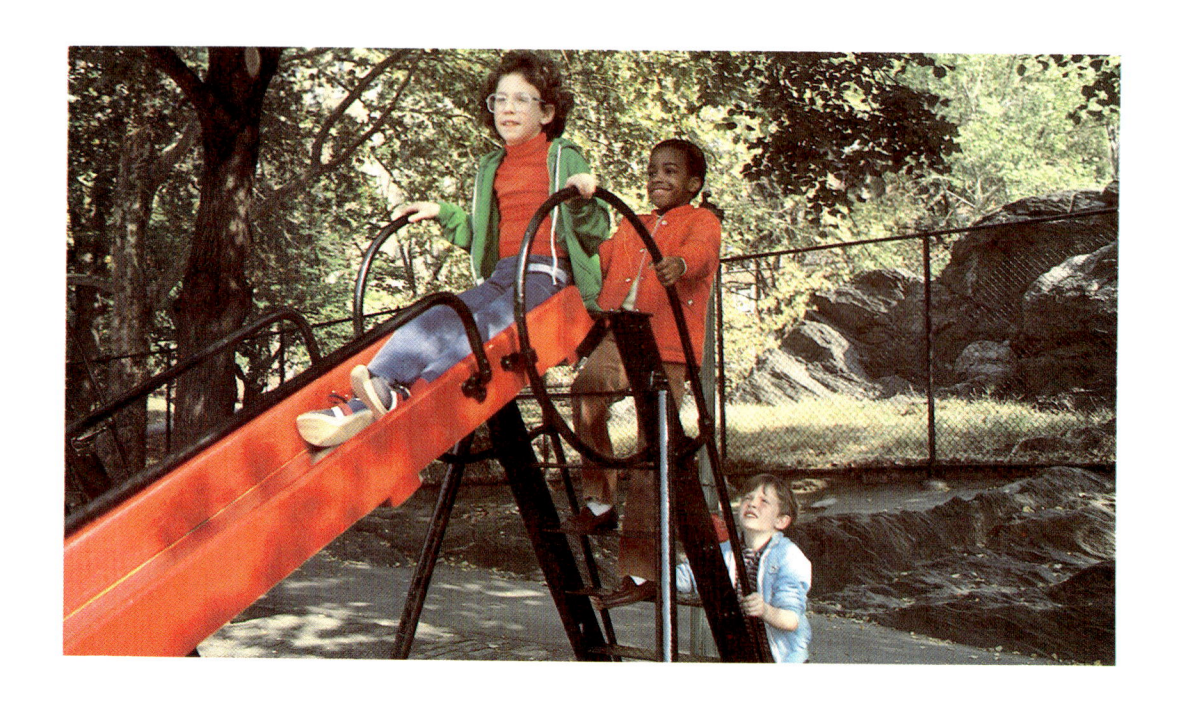

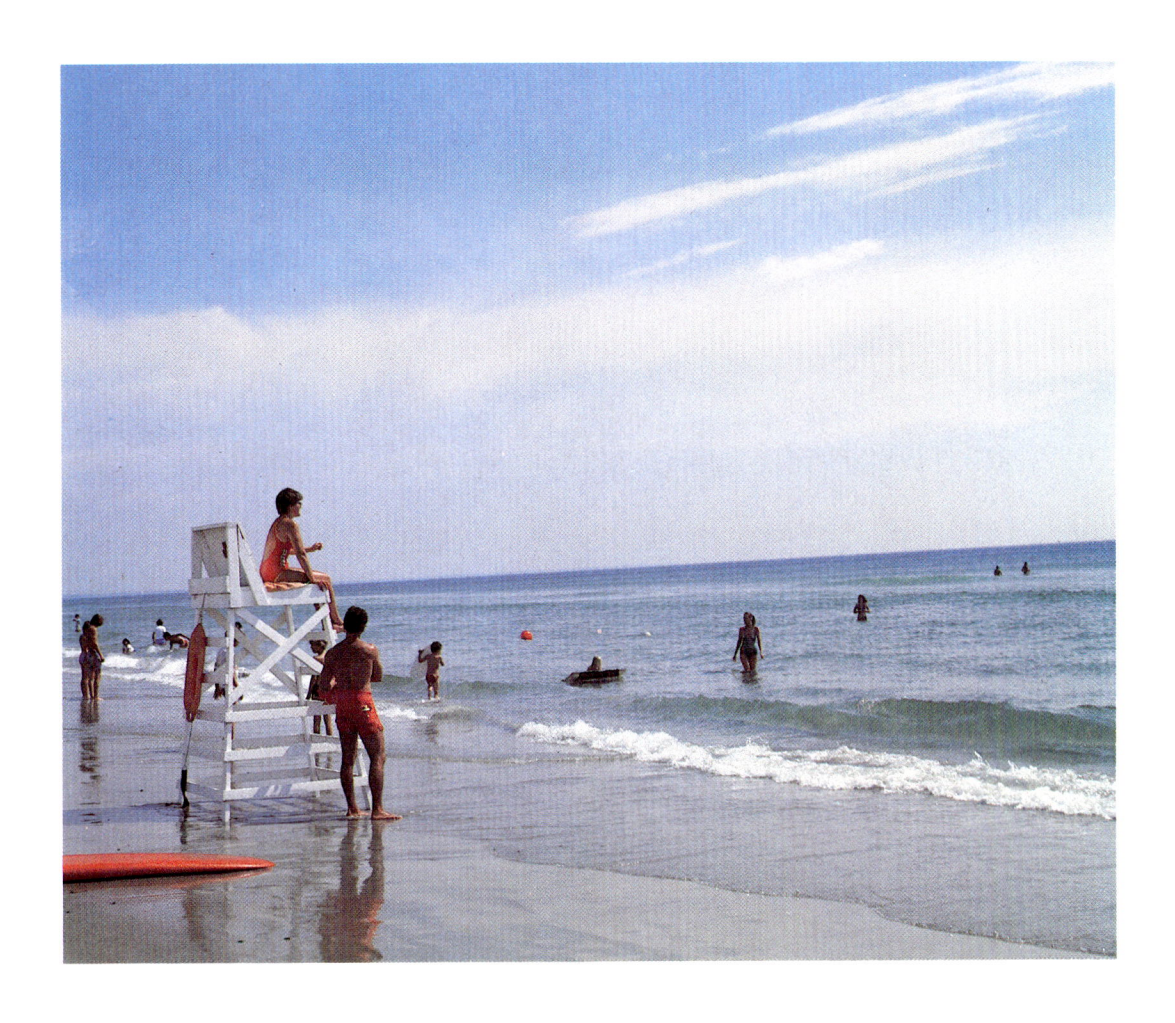

Look at both pictures.

Tell how the children are watching out for their safety.

Name some other safety rules for playing outside.

Tell how to help keep accidents from happening.

Safety Inside

Most accidents happen at home. Someone may slip on a wet floor. Someone may trip over things that are left on the floor. Wipe up spills as soon as you see them. Put away your toys. Don't leave things on stairs.

Do your part to help keep accidents from happening. Make safety a habit.

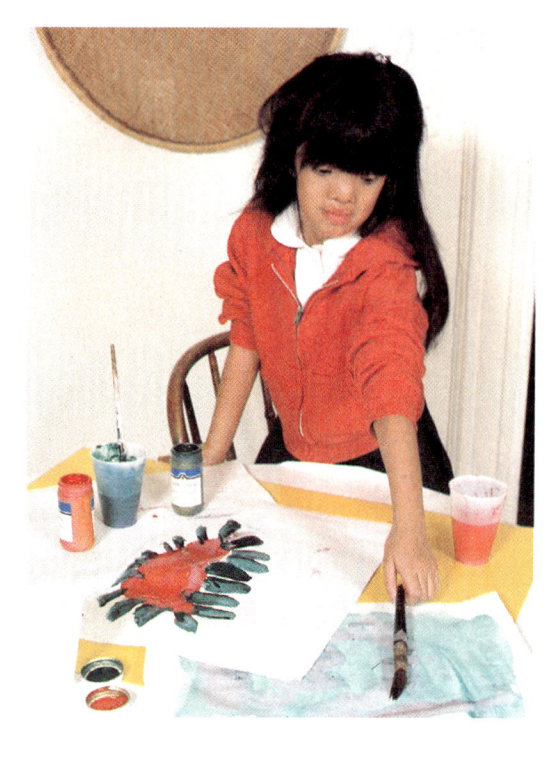

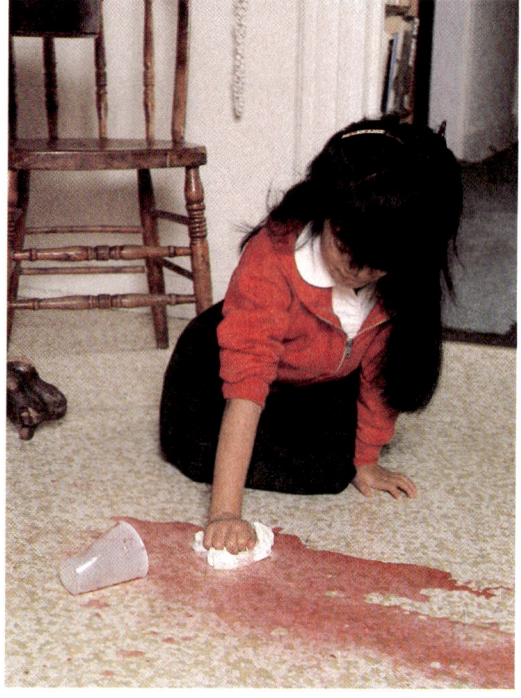

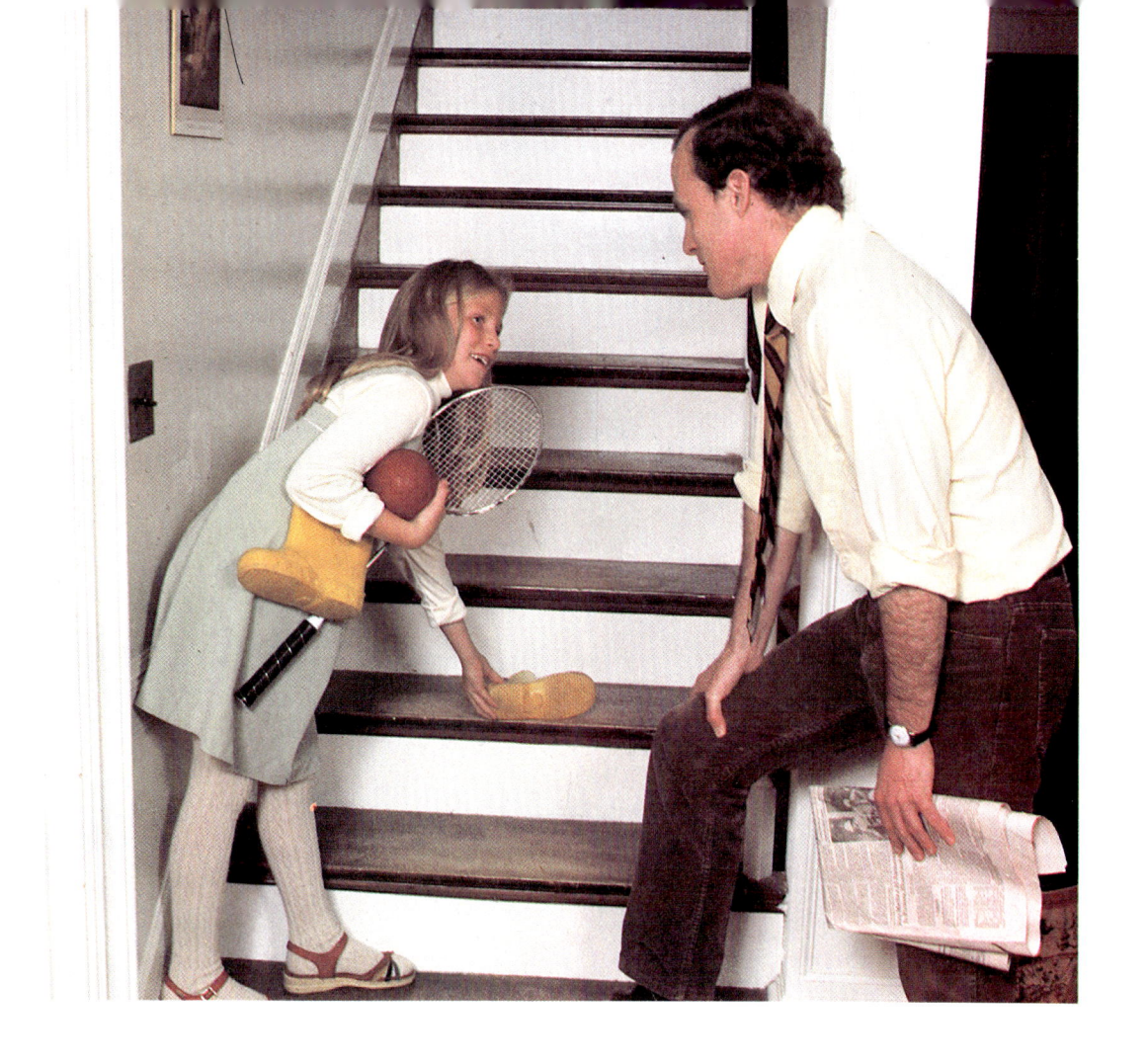

Look at the pictures on page 144.

Is the girl doing her part to help keep accidents from happening?

How can you tell?

Look at the picture on this page.

What is the girl doing to help keep accidents from happening?

What are some other good safety habits?

145

When Accidents Happen

Sometimes accidents happen. Stay calm. Act quickly. Get help from a grown-up.

First aid is a kind of help. A scrape may need first aid. Wash the scrape. Clean dirt and germs away. Then, cover it to keep it clean. Learn first aid for other injuries. Learn about other helpful things to do when accidents happen.

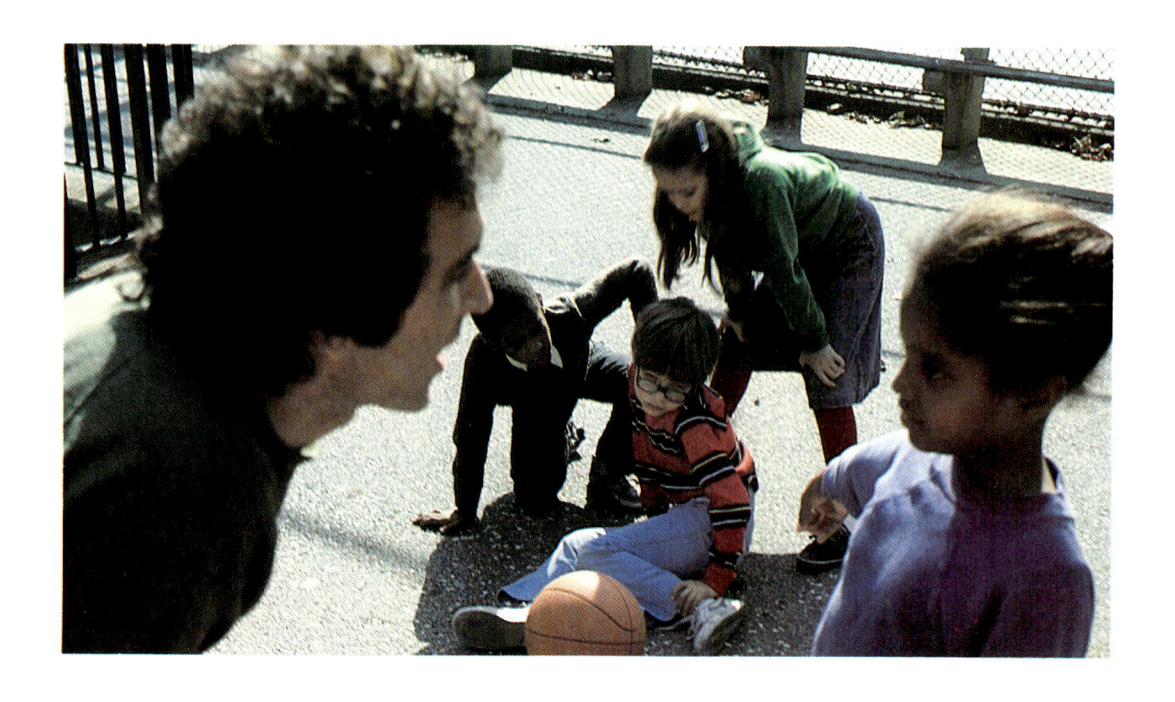

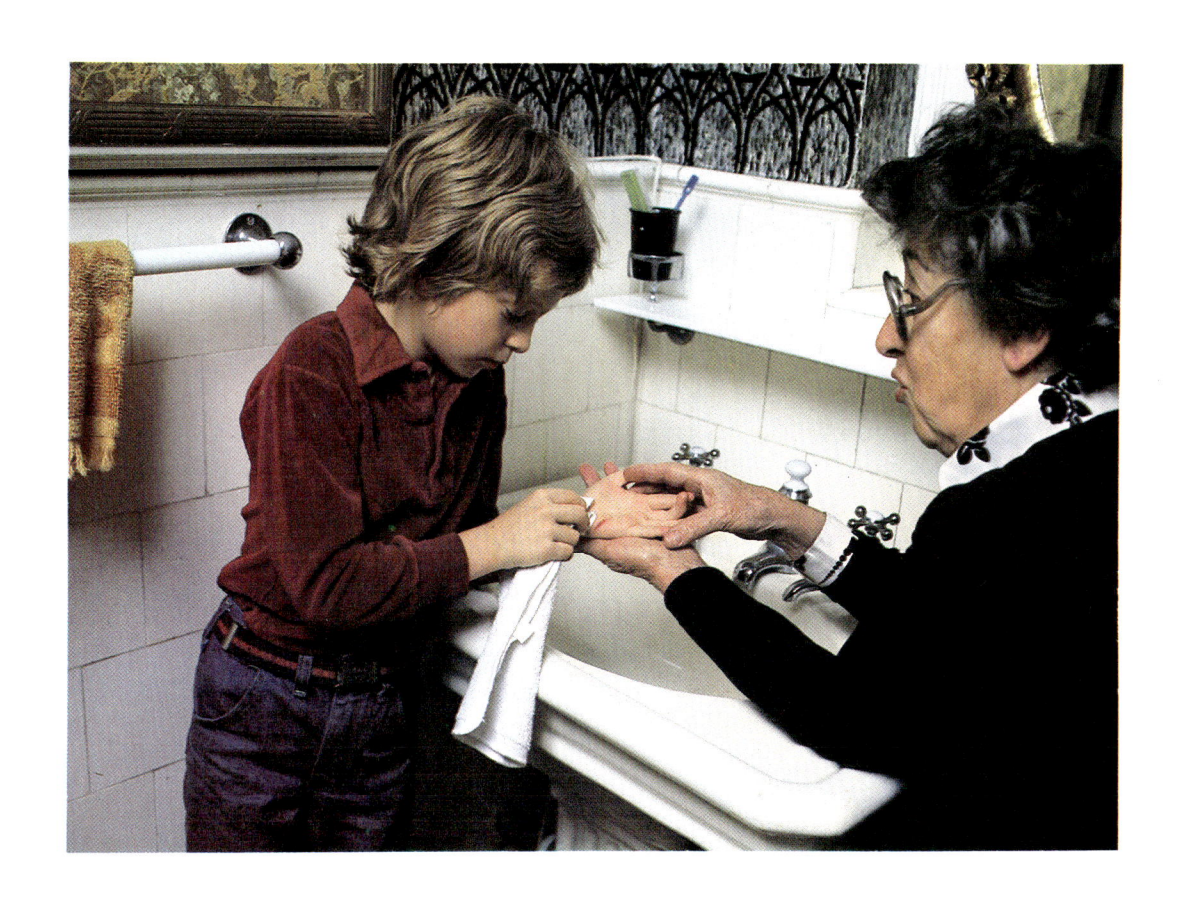

Look at the picture on page 146.

What may have happened?

Whom is the girl telling?

Why is it important to tell a grown-up?

Look at the picture on this page.

What may have happened to this boy?

What kind of help is he getting?

What should you do after an accident?

Your Turn

A Stray Dog

Karen is on her way to school. She sees a dog. The dog is walking toward her. It doesn't seem to have an owner, but it does seem to be friendly.

Help Karen.
Tell what she should do.
Tell why she should do it.

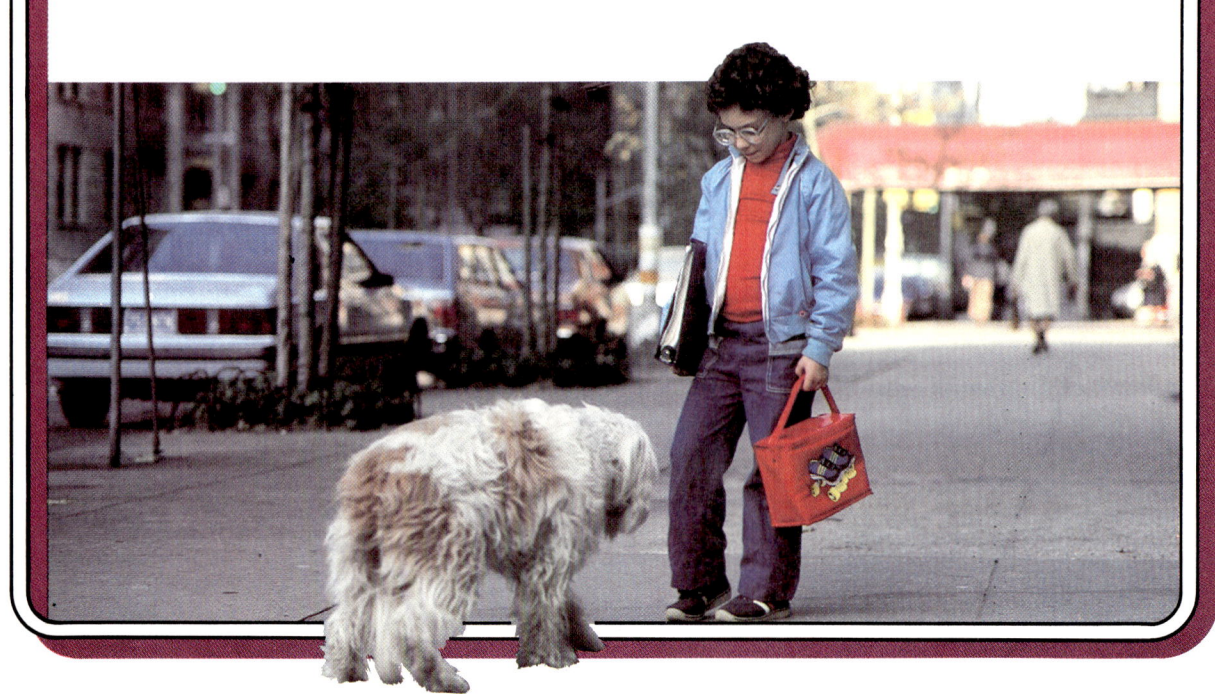

Health in Action

1. Draw a picture. Show a place where you can play a running game safely.

2. Make believe you are on a bus trip. Tell about some safety rules. Tell what you could do to have fun.

3. Make a first-aid kit. Keep it handy.

4. Make a poster. List some safety rules for home. Show the poster to your family. Try to work together to help keep accidents from happening.

Do You Remember?

Your Health Words

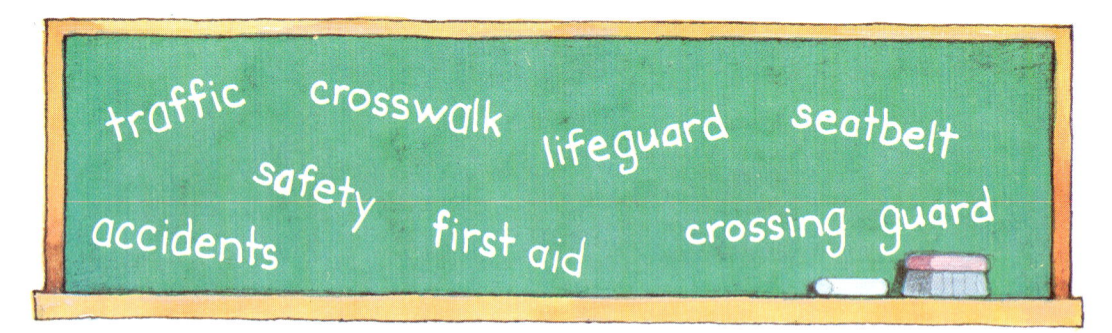

traffic crosswalk lifeguard seatbelt safety accidents first aid crossing guard

Answer the questions.

Use the Health Words.

1. Where can you cross a street safely?
2. What helps with safety in a car?
3. Who helps with safety around water?

Your Health Ideas

1. List some rules for bicycle safety.
2. Tell how to ride safely in buses and cars.
3. Name some habits for safety outside.
4. Name some habits for safety at home.

Health Check-Up

Tell which sentences are true.

1. You should cross a street at the corner.
2. It helps to stay calm after an accident.
3. You should ride a bicycle next to someone else.
4. You should stay seated when in a bus.
5. It is safe to tease animals.
6. You should swim alone.
7. It is safe to play running games near swings and slides.
8. A scrape needs first aid.
9. You should wipe up spills.
10. A seatbelt can help keep you safe in a car.

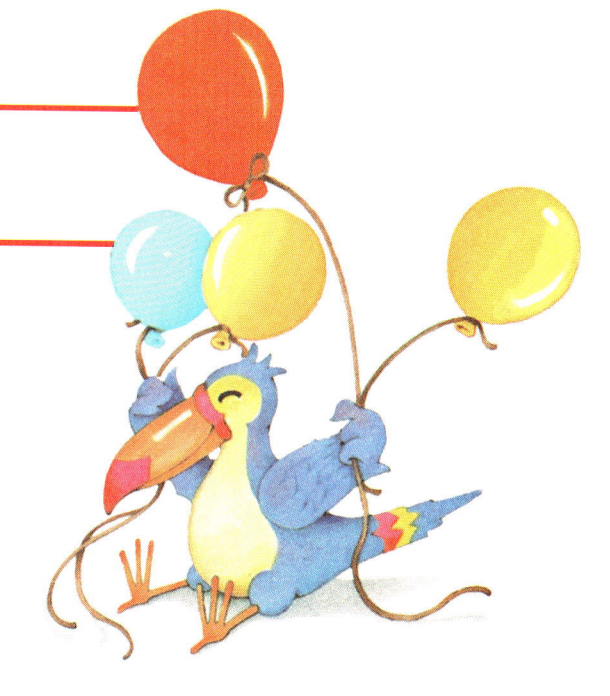

CHAPTER 8

The World Around You

Your world is where you work and play. It is where you sleep and eat. It is a special place. Treat it as you would treat anything that is special. Take care of it. Help keep it quiet, clean, and safe. Help keep it a healthful place to live.

What can you do to help take care of your world?

Health Words

environment
natural resources
energy
electricity

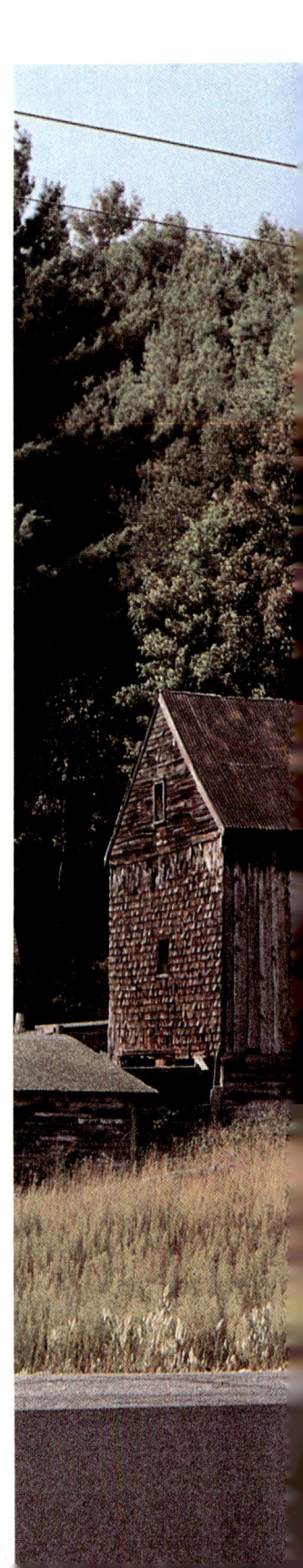

water
pollution
litter

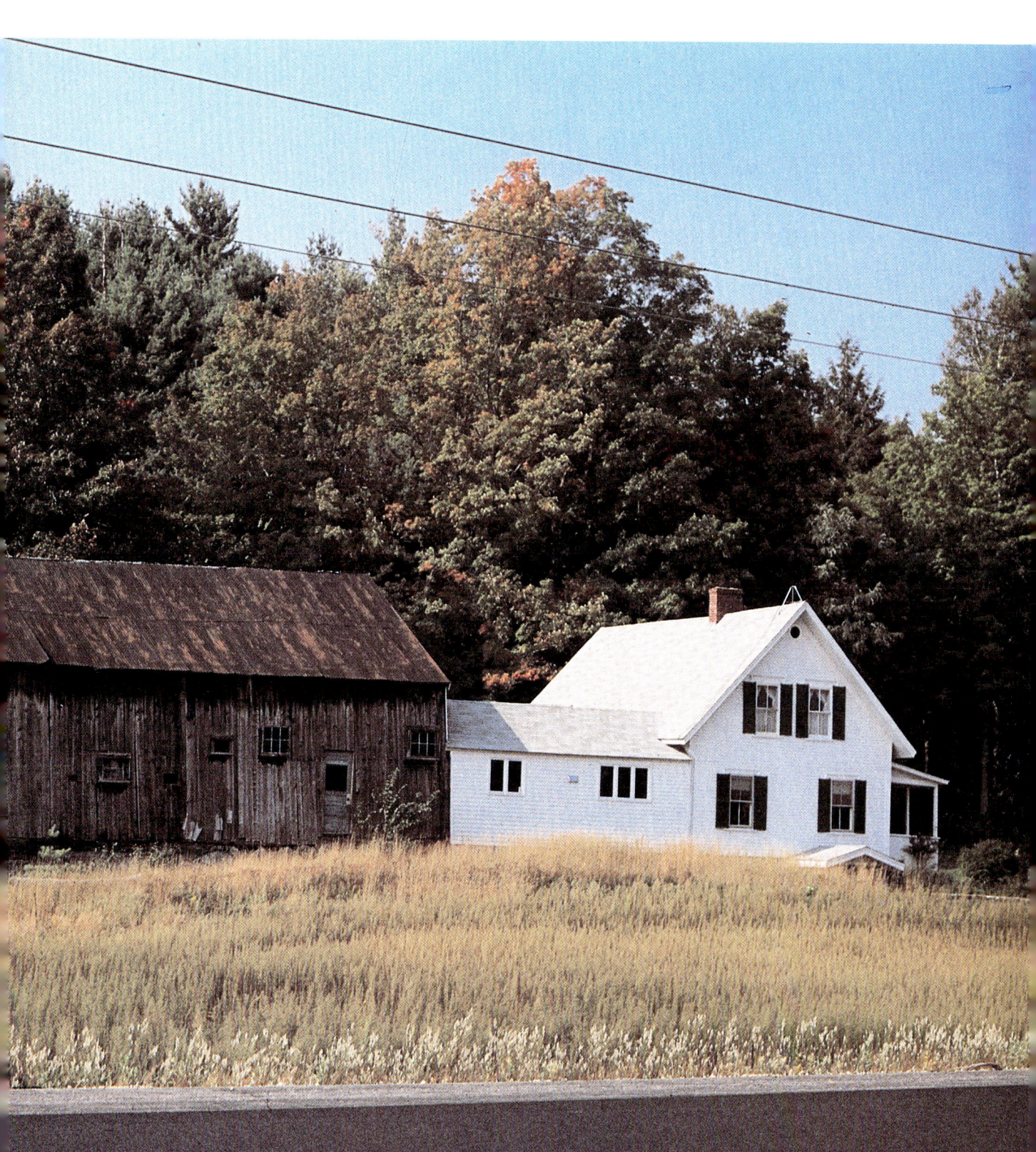

Helping Your World

Your environment is your world. It is made up of everything around you. You share your environment with others. You and others can help take care of it. You can work together. You can help the world around you stay clean and healthful.

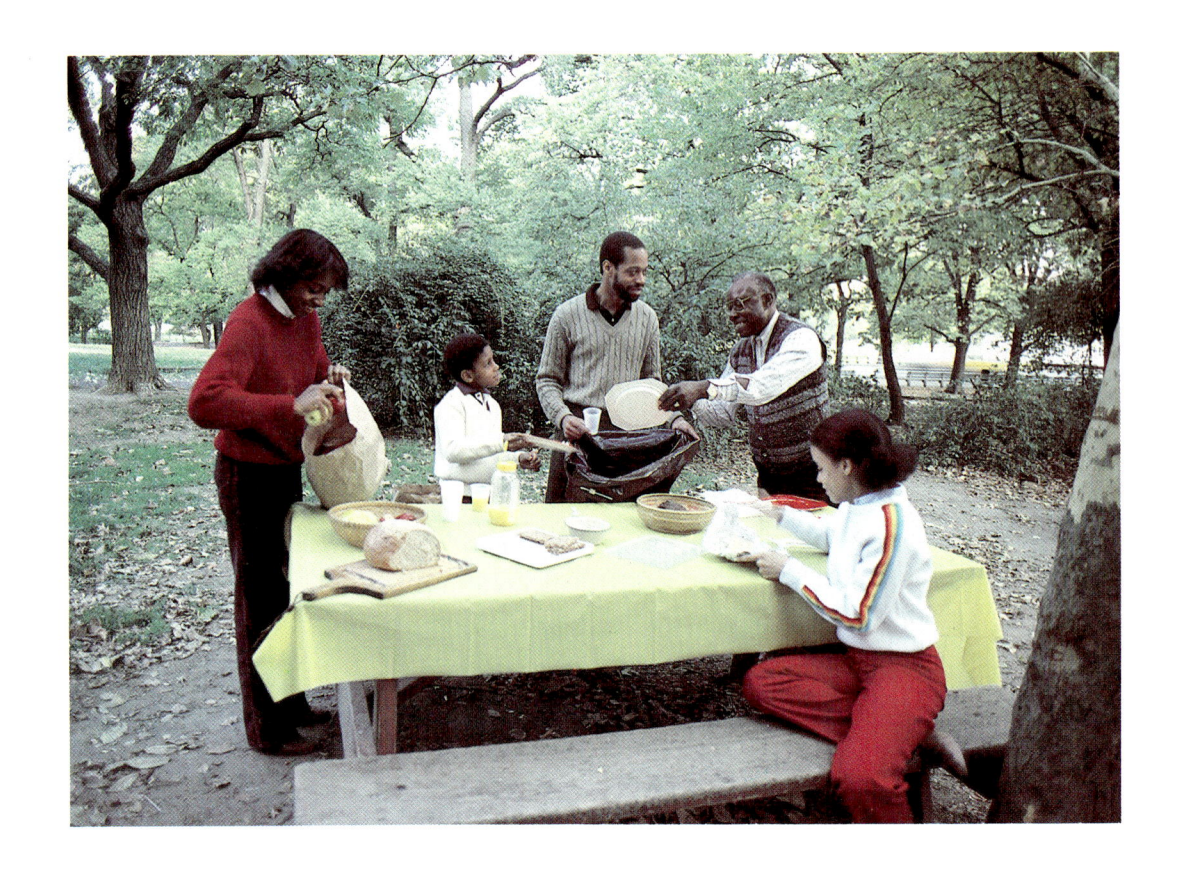

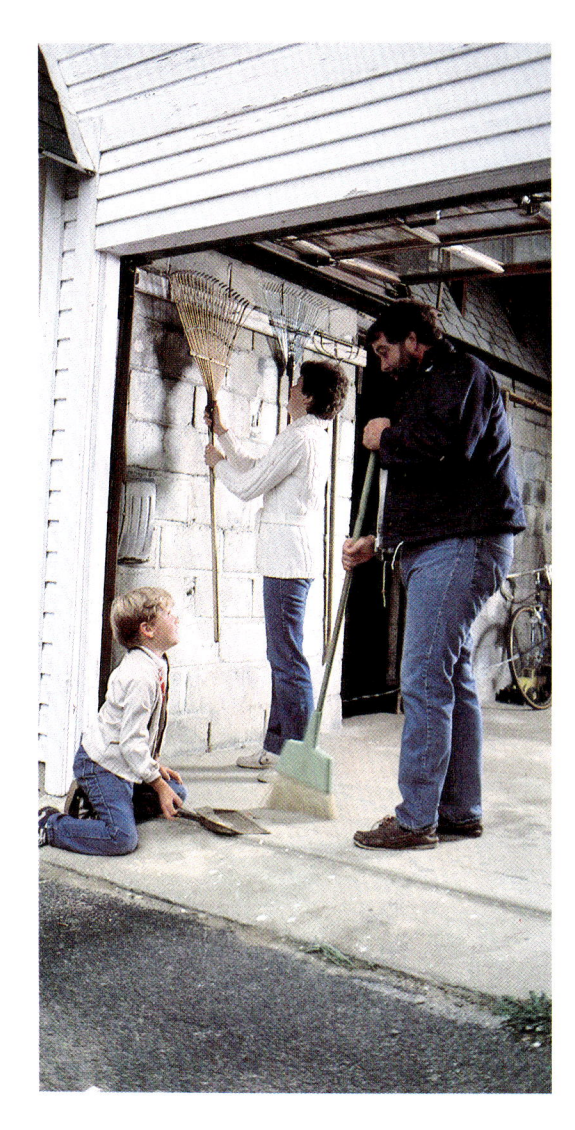

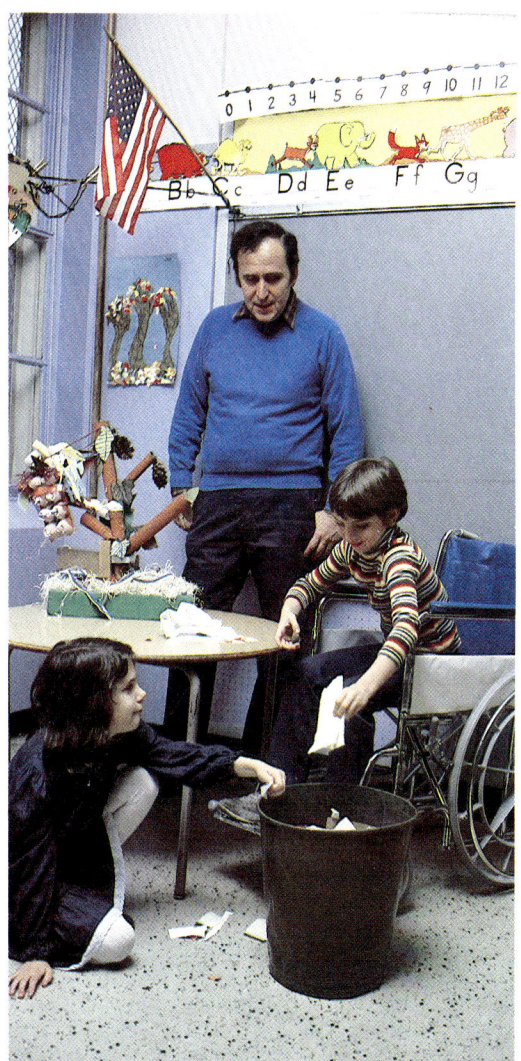

Look at all three pictures.

How are the people helping to take care of their environment?

Tell about some other ways to help.

Tell why helping is important.

155

Saving Energy

Coal and oil are natural resources. They are used to make energy. Energy is used to make electricity. Electricity is used in many ways. You use electricity every time you turn on a light.

There is only so much coal and oil in the earth, and no more. Help save these natural resources. Help save energy. Do not waste electricity.

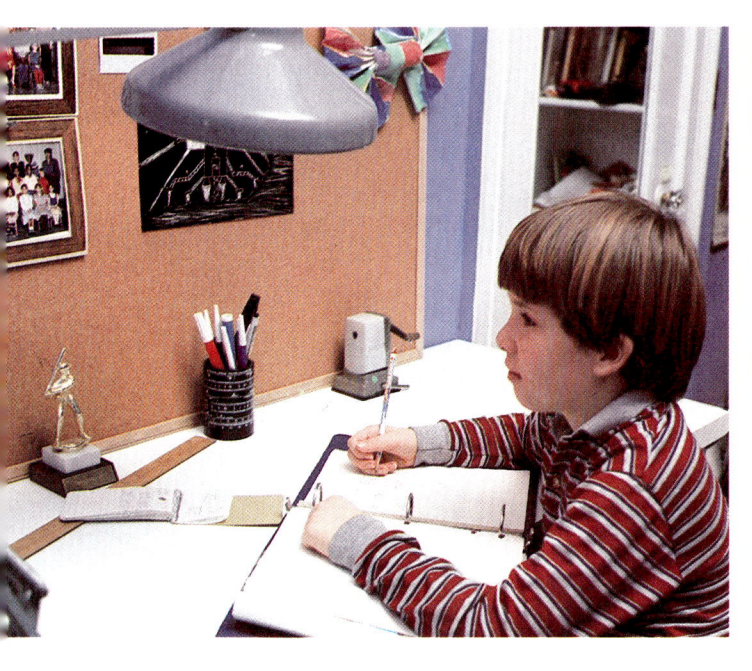

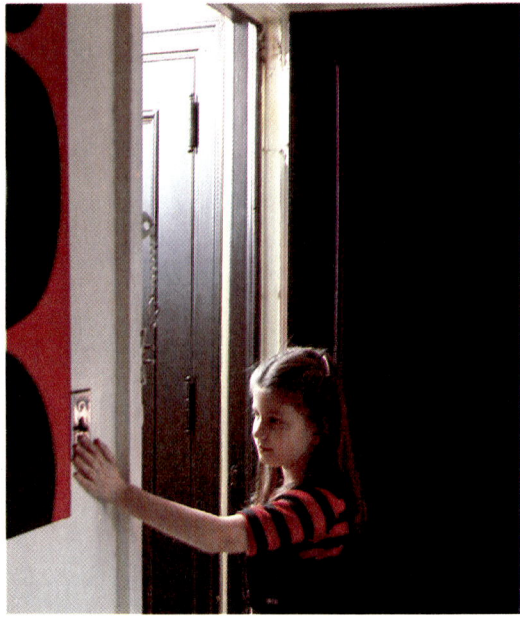

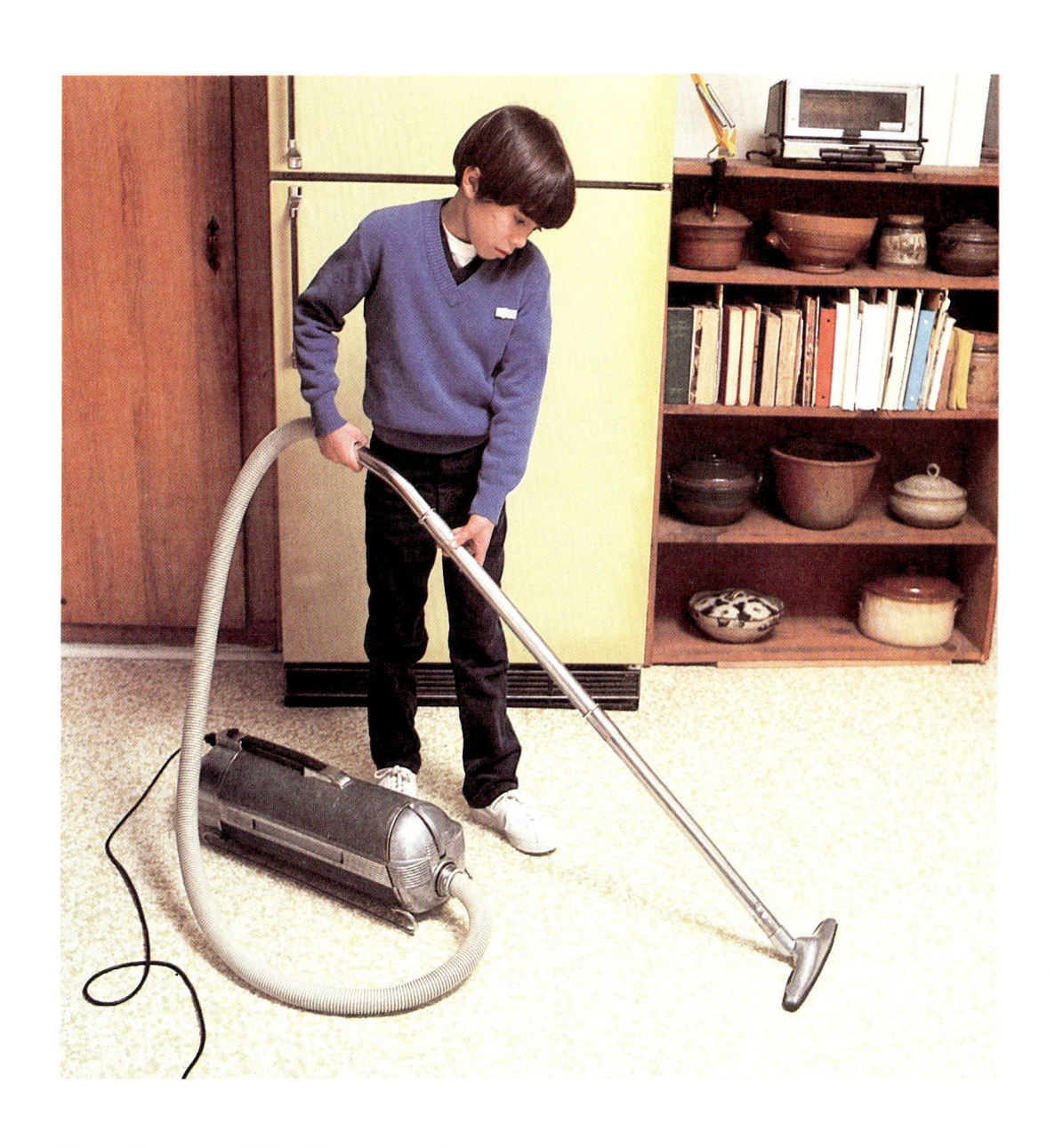

Look at all three pictures.

Which things use electricity?

What is the girl doing to help save energy?

Tell some other ways to help save energy.

Saving Paper and Water

Trees and water are important natural resources. The wood in trees is used to make different kinds of paper. We use paper every day. We use water every day, too. We need water to live and stay healthy.

Help save these important natural resources. Use both sides of every sheet of paper. Use only the water you need.

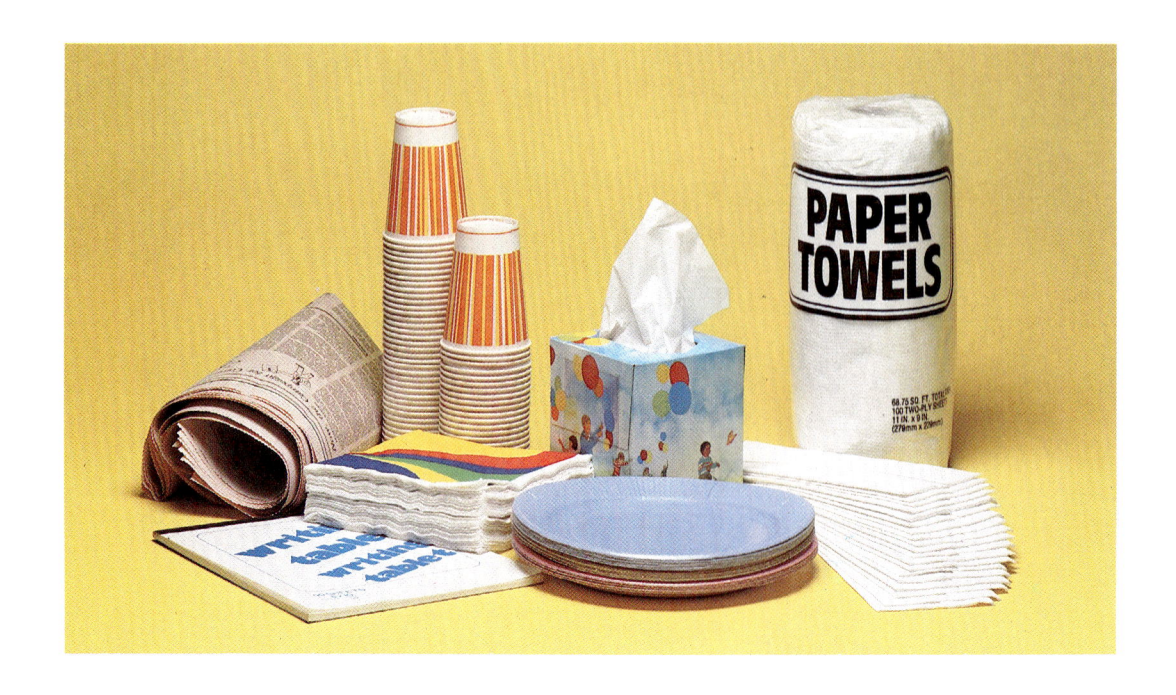

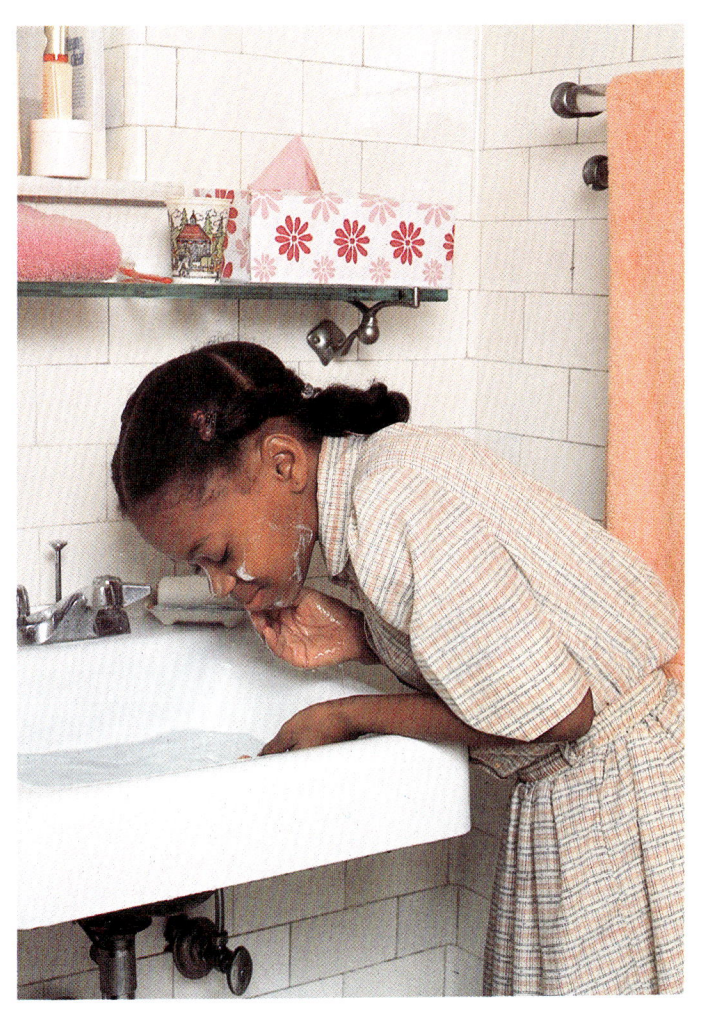

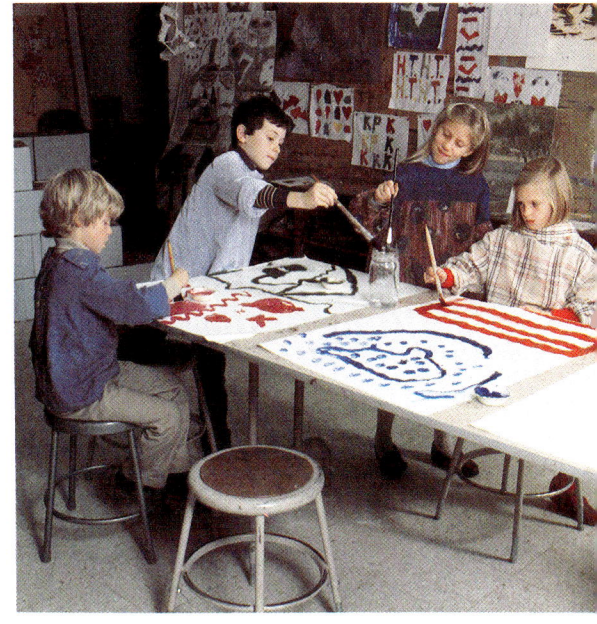

Look at the picture on page 158.
Name the things made from paper.
How can you help save paper?

Look at the pictures on this page.
How are the children saving water?
What else can you do to save water?

Using Things Again

A shoebox can hold other things besides shoes. The same is true for many things. Before you throw away something, look at it. Ask yourself, "Can I use this in another way?"

There are many ways to help save our natural resources. Doing your part can be fun.

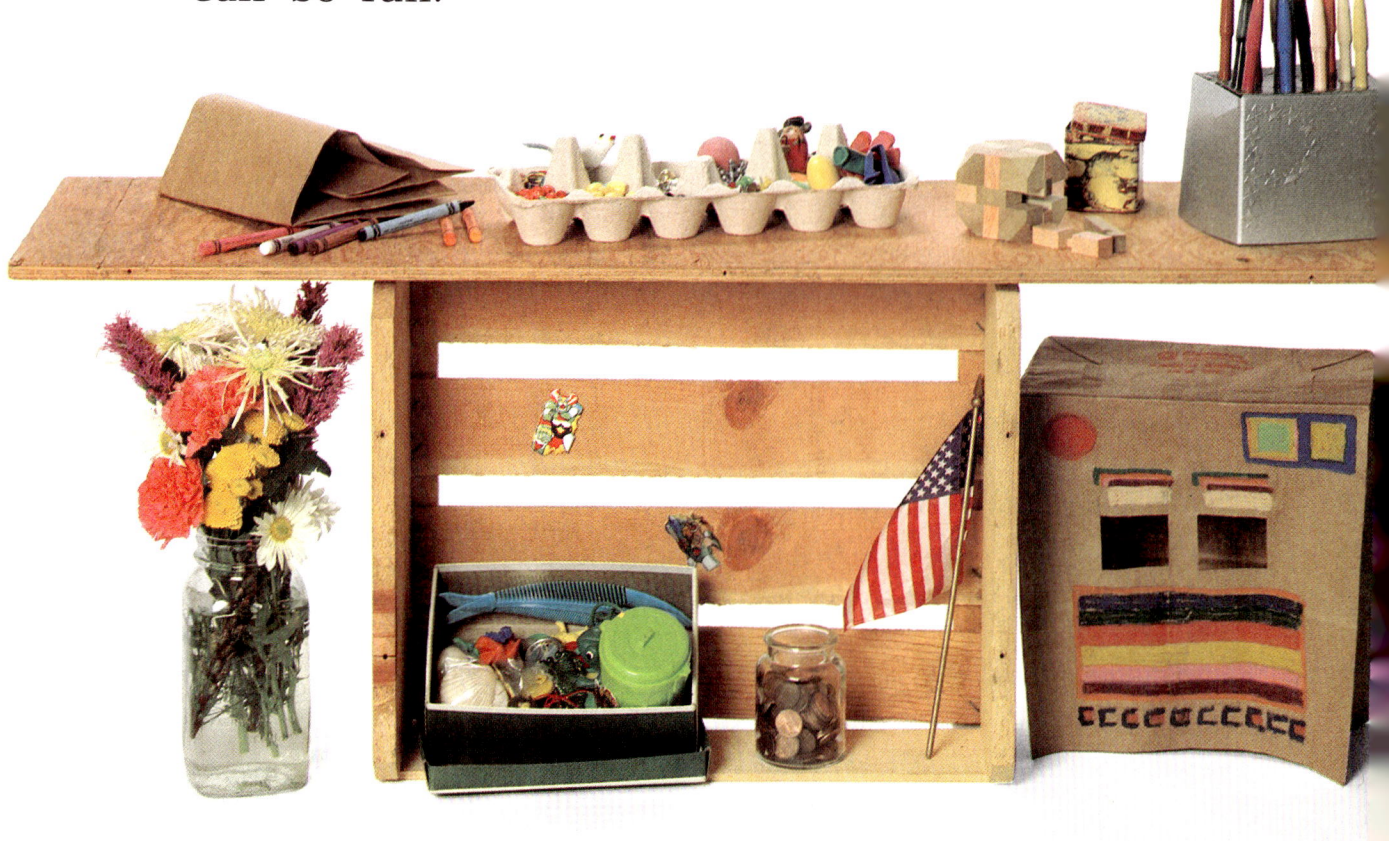

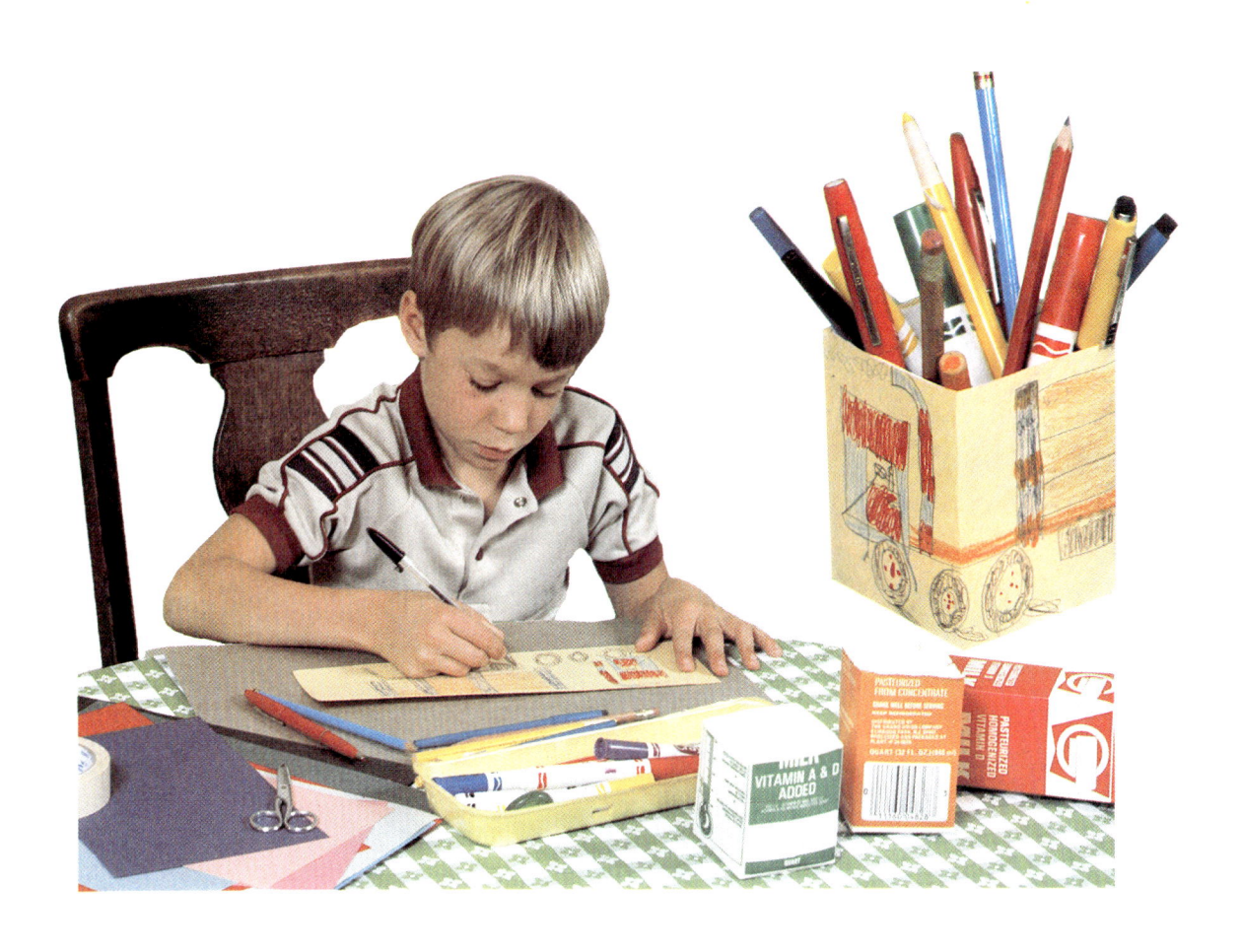

Look at the things on page 160.
Tell what was used to make each thing.

Look at the pictures on this page.
What is the boy using to make a pencil holder?

What other things can be used again?
Tell how they can be used.
Tell how using things again can help save our natural resources.

Health Highlight

Junk Art

Jean Tinguely is a kind of artist. He does not use paint and brushes. He makes his art from junk.

He uses things other people might throw away. He puts them together in new ways. He turns them into art. Some people like his art.

What do you think about his art?

What else can you do with junk besides throw it away?

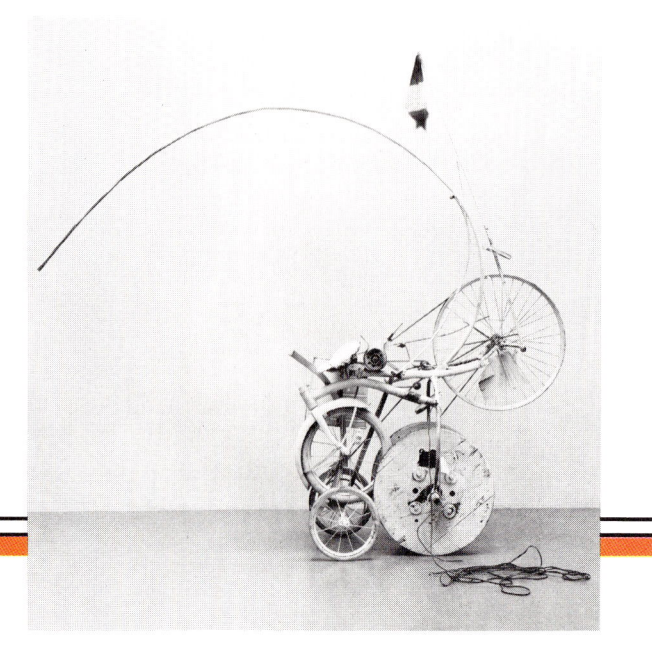

Going, Seeing, and Doing

1. Go into different rooms at home. Find things made from paper. Make a list of the things. Then, tell how you can help save paper.

2. Watch other people. Are they helping to save our natural resources? How? What can you do to help?

3. Find some things at home that are not used anymore. Ask if you can bring them to school. Use them to make a piece of art.

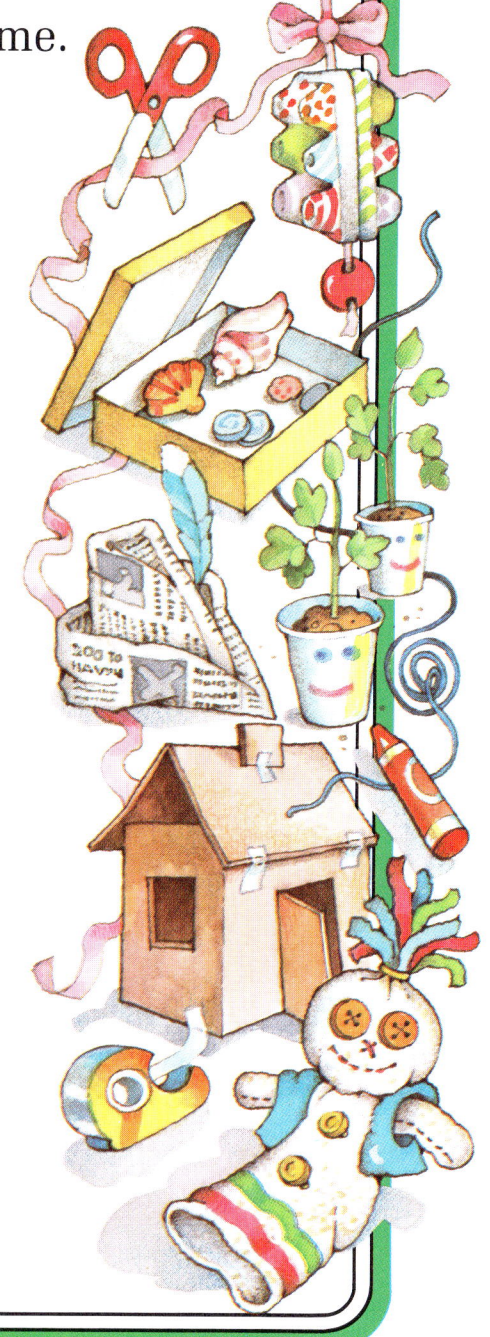

The Noise Around You

Pollution is anything that harms the environment. Noise can be a kind of pollution. When noise is too loud, it can be harmful.

Try to stay away from loud machines. Cover your ears when you can't. Keep radios and TVs turned down low. Protect your hearing from harmful noise.

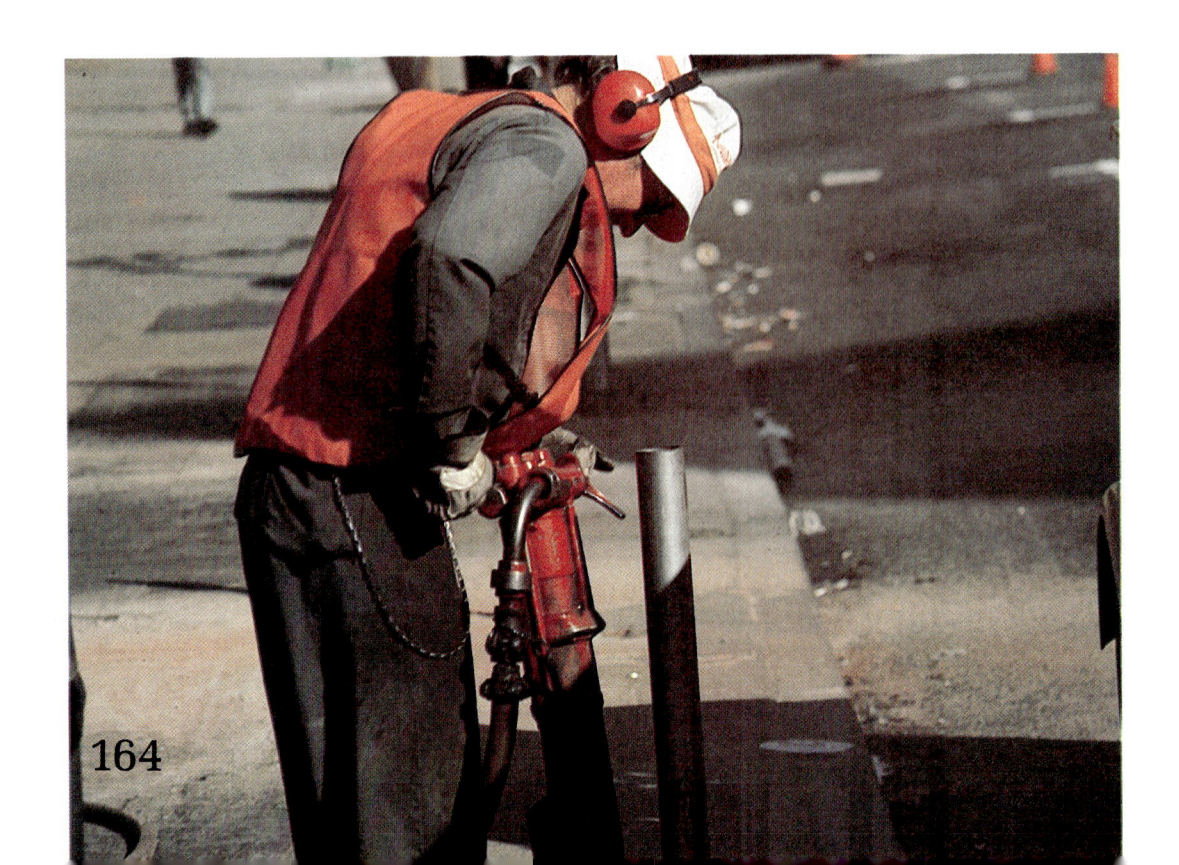

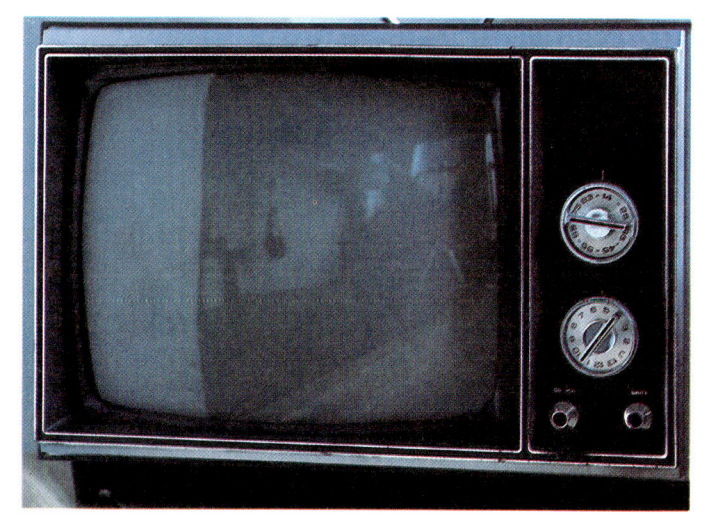

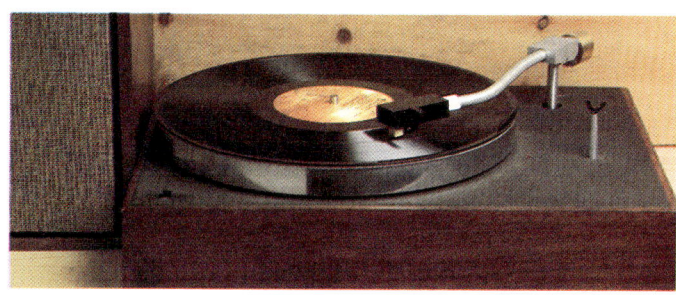

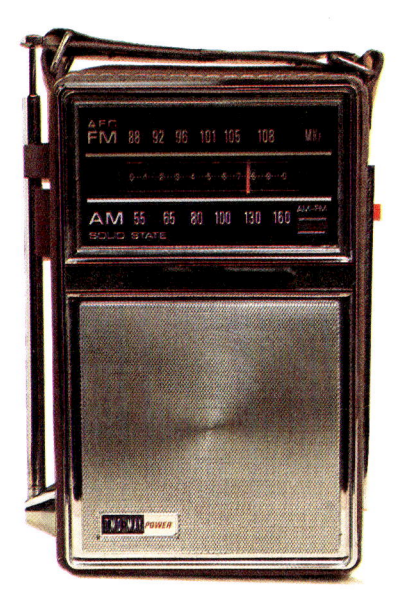

Look at the picture on page 164.

How is the worker helping to protect his ears?

Look at the pictures on this page.

How can you protect your hearing when you use these things?

What else can you do to protect your hearing?

165

Helping to Care for the Outdoors

Litter is a kind of pollution. It makes the outdoors dirty. It makes the outdoors ugly. Litter can be harmful.

Don't litter. Throw trash in a trash can. Clean up after picnics. Clean up after playing outside. It feels good to have a clean outdoors. It feels good to do your part.

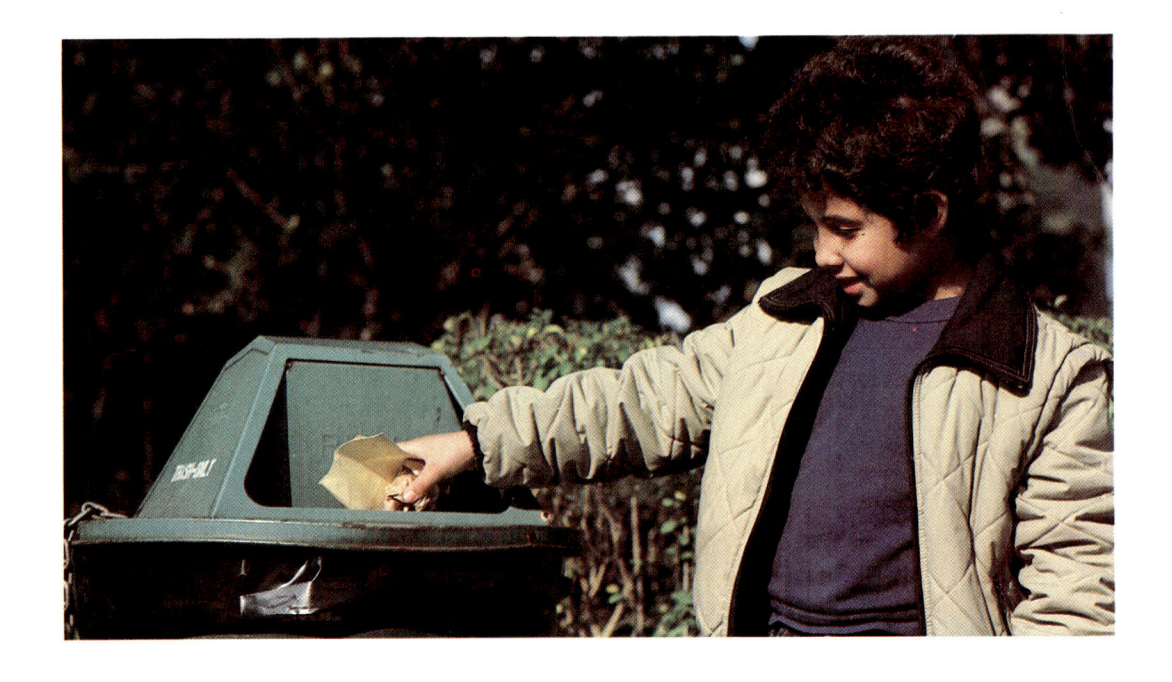

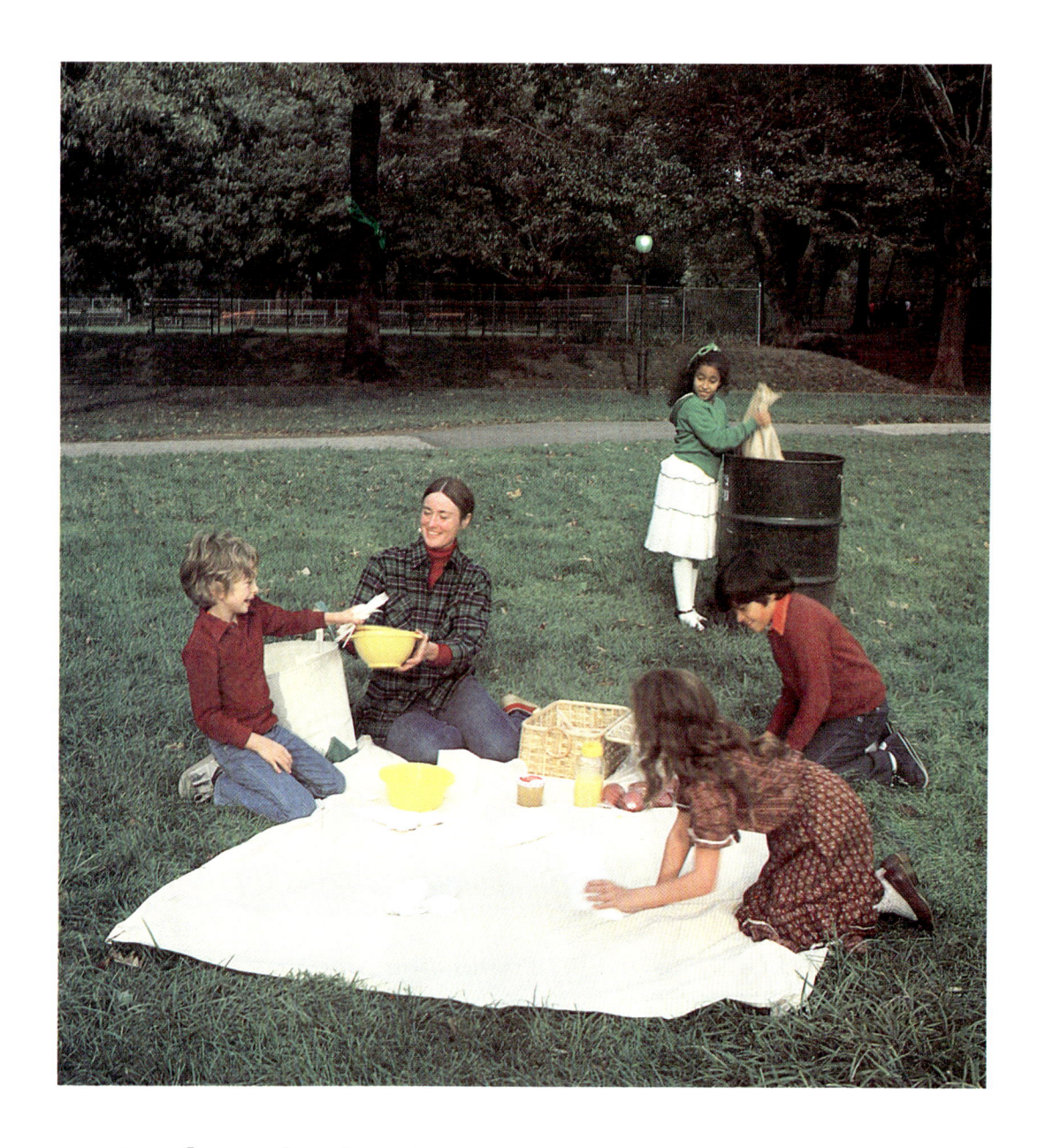

Look at both pictures.

How are the children helping to take care of the outdoors?

Tell some other ways to help.

Helping to Care for Your Home

You can feel proud of a home that is neat and clean. Do your part to help. Take care of your things. Help keep them looking nice. Put things back where they belong. Help others in your family do the same.

Your home is part of your environment. Help take care of it.

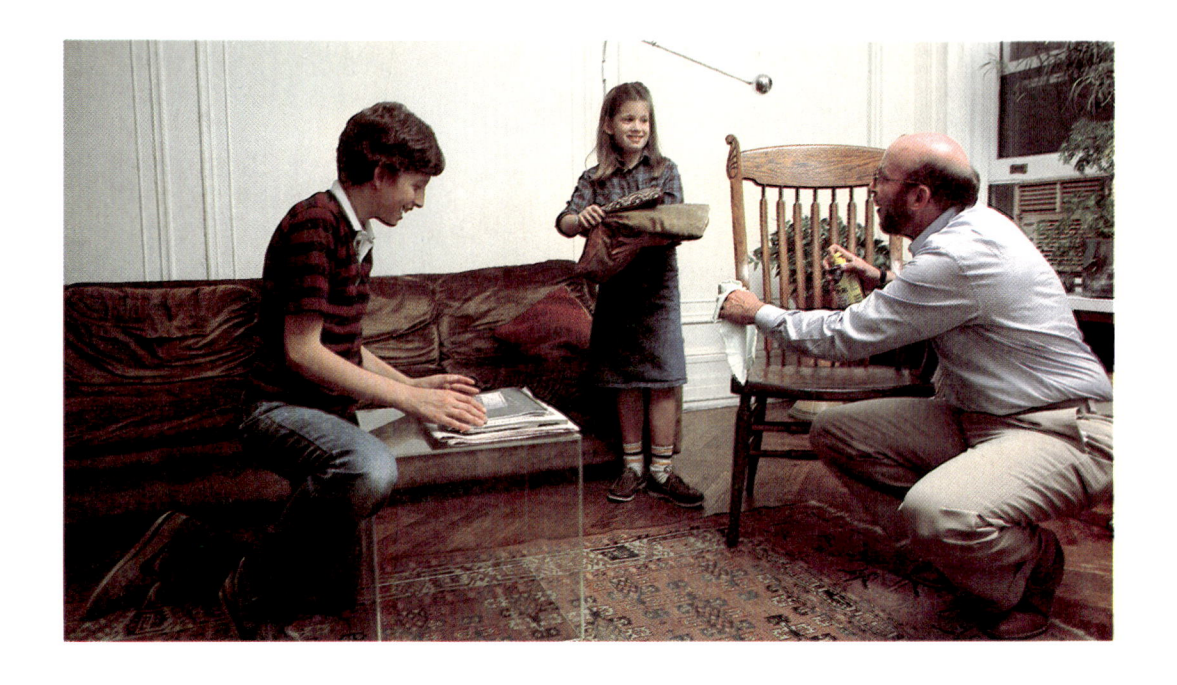

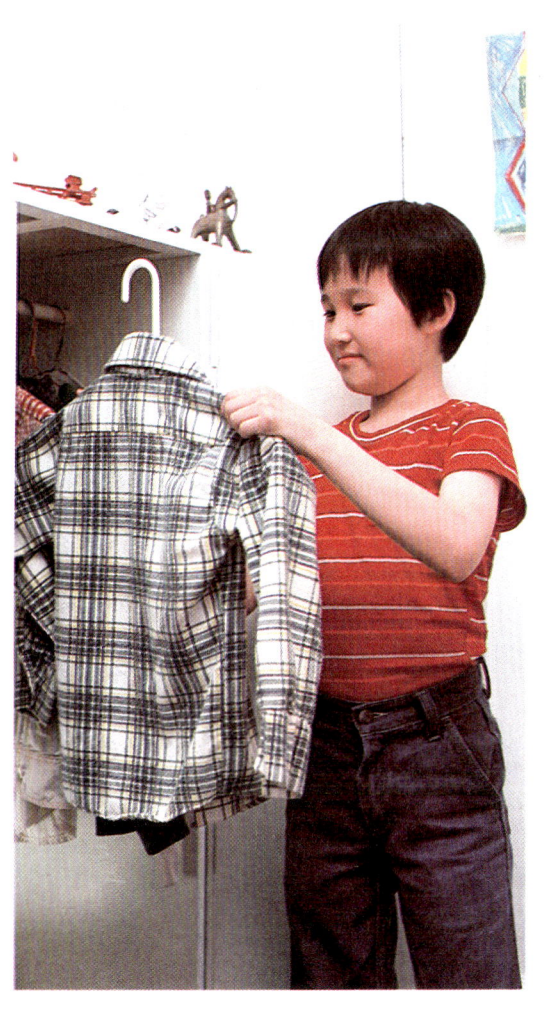

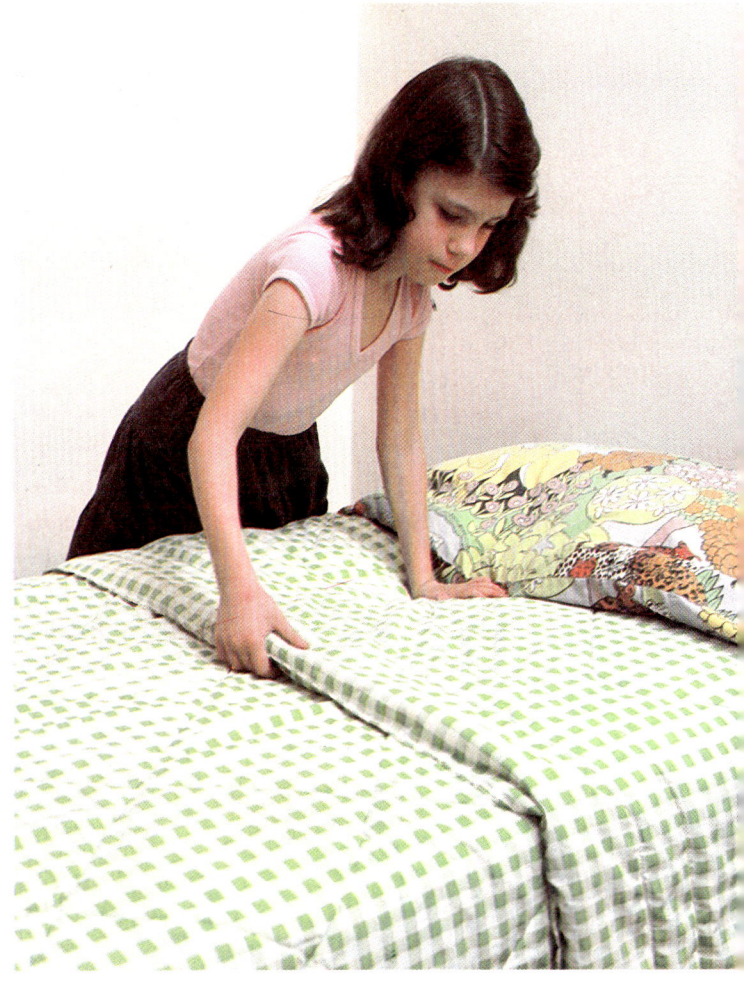

Look at all three pictures.

How are the people helping to take care of their homes?

Tell some other ways to help.

Tell why helping in these ways is important.

169

Your Turn

The Gift Box

Jason got some books. They came in a big, strong box. He looked at the box. He couldn't decide what to do with it.

Help Jason.

What can he do with the box?

Tell how your ideas could help save our natural resources.

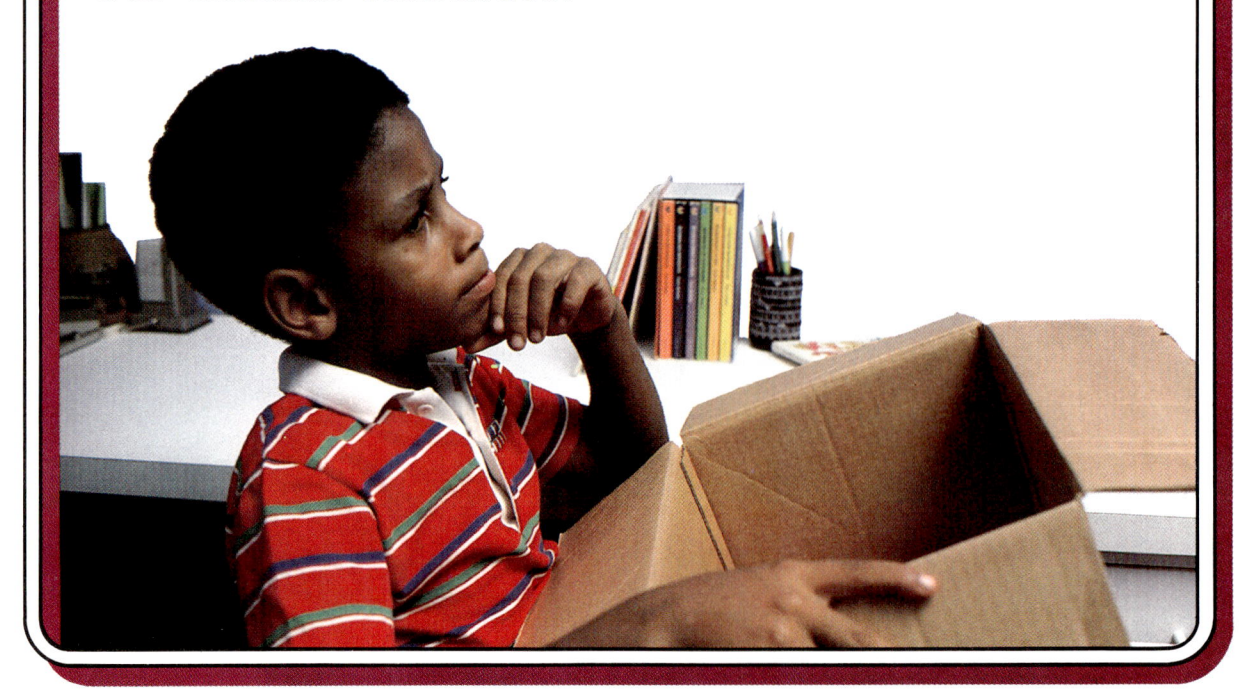

Health in Action

1. Name some things that make noise. How can you protect your ears from noise pollution?

2. Ask a grown-up in your family for an empty box. Use the box to make something you can use.

3. What can you do to help keep your home neat and clean? Make a list. Do the things on the list.

4. Water is a natural resource. It has many uses. Find out about some of them. Make a list. Talk about your list in class.

Do You Remember?

Your Health Words

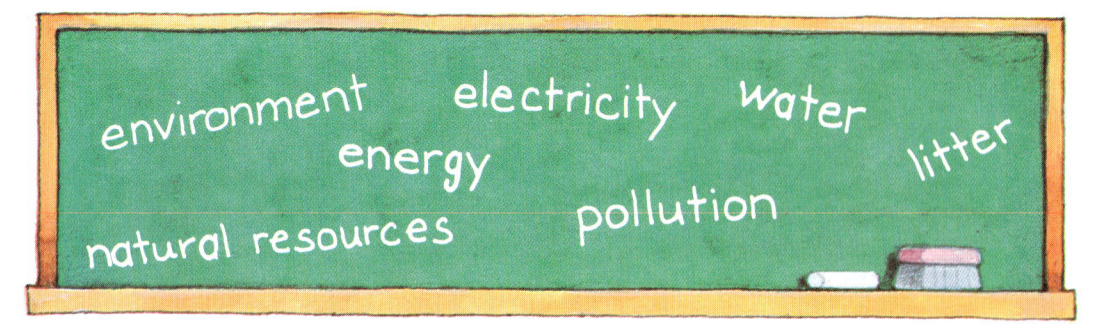

environment   electricity   water
energy
litter
natural resources   pollution

Finish the sentences.

Use the Health Words.

1. Trees are one of our ____.
2. Noise ____ can harm your ears.
3. You can help keep your ____ clean.

Your Health Ideas

1. Tell why saving energy is important.
2. List some ways to help save paper.
3. Tell why litter is harmful.
4. Tell how to help care for the outdoors.

Health Check-Up

Tell which sentences are true.

1. You share your environment with others.
2. There are ways to save electricity.
3. Trees are not a natural resource.
4. You should always throw away paper after using one side.
5. It can be fun to help save our natural resources.
6. Trash belongs on the ground.
7. Noise pollution can harm your ears.
8. Litter helps to make the outdoors beautiful.
9. Pollution helps the environment.
10. You can help take care of your home.

Exercise Handbook

This part of your book is about exercise. You need exercise every day. It helps you stay healthy. It helps you look and feel good. Ask your doctor which exercises are best for you.

Stretching Out

When you exercise, begin by stretching your muscles. Stretching helps get your muscles ready for other exercises. It helps protect them from injury. It helps make them strong.

sky stretches

straddle stretches

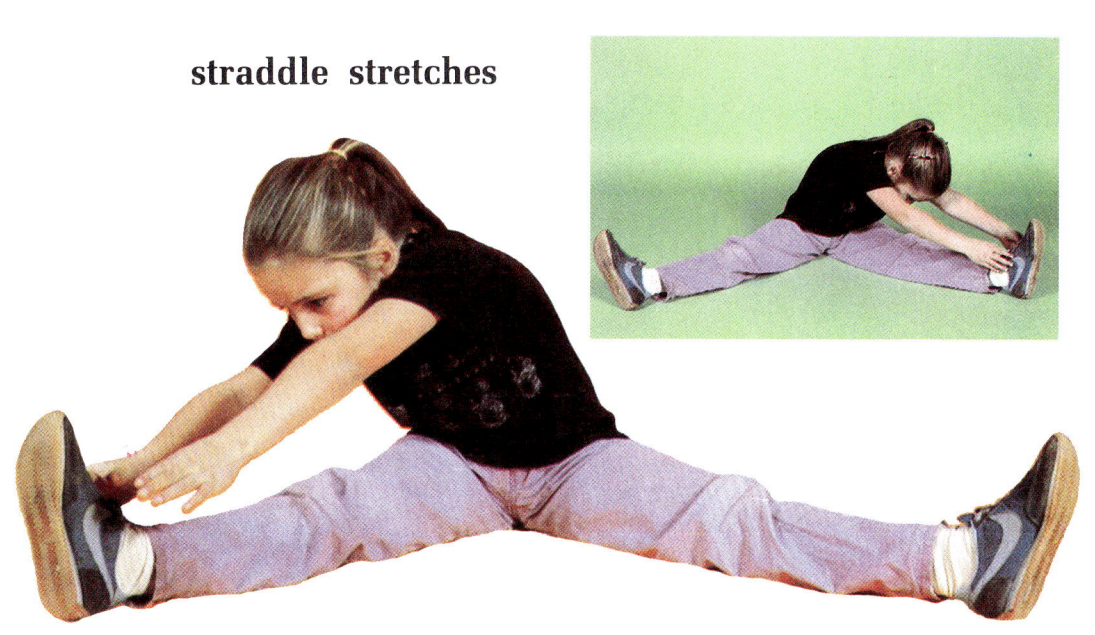

thigh stretches

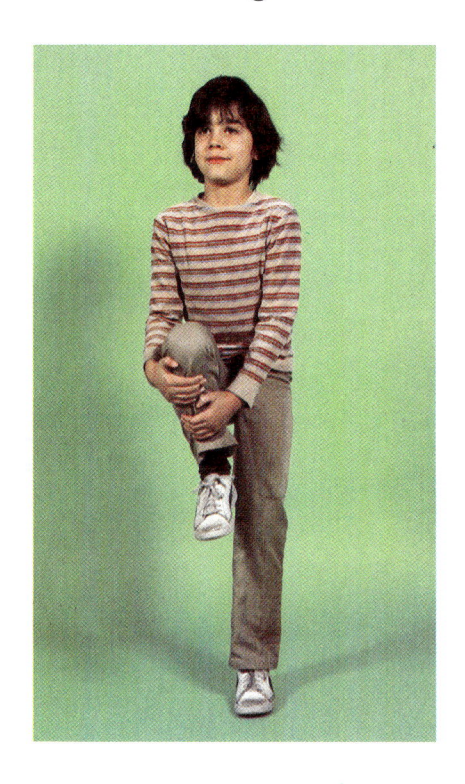

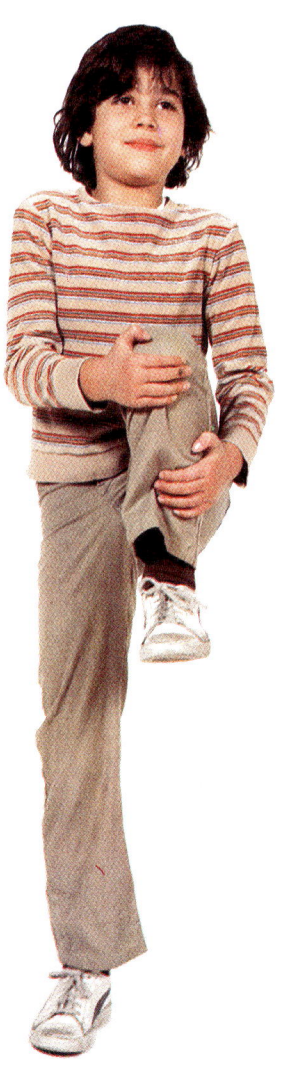

Having Fun with Movement

You can do some exercises by yourself. You can do some with others. You can have fun when you exercise.

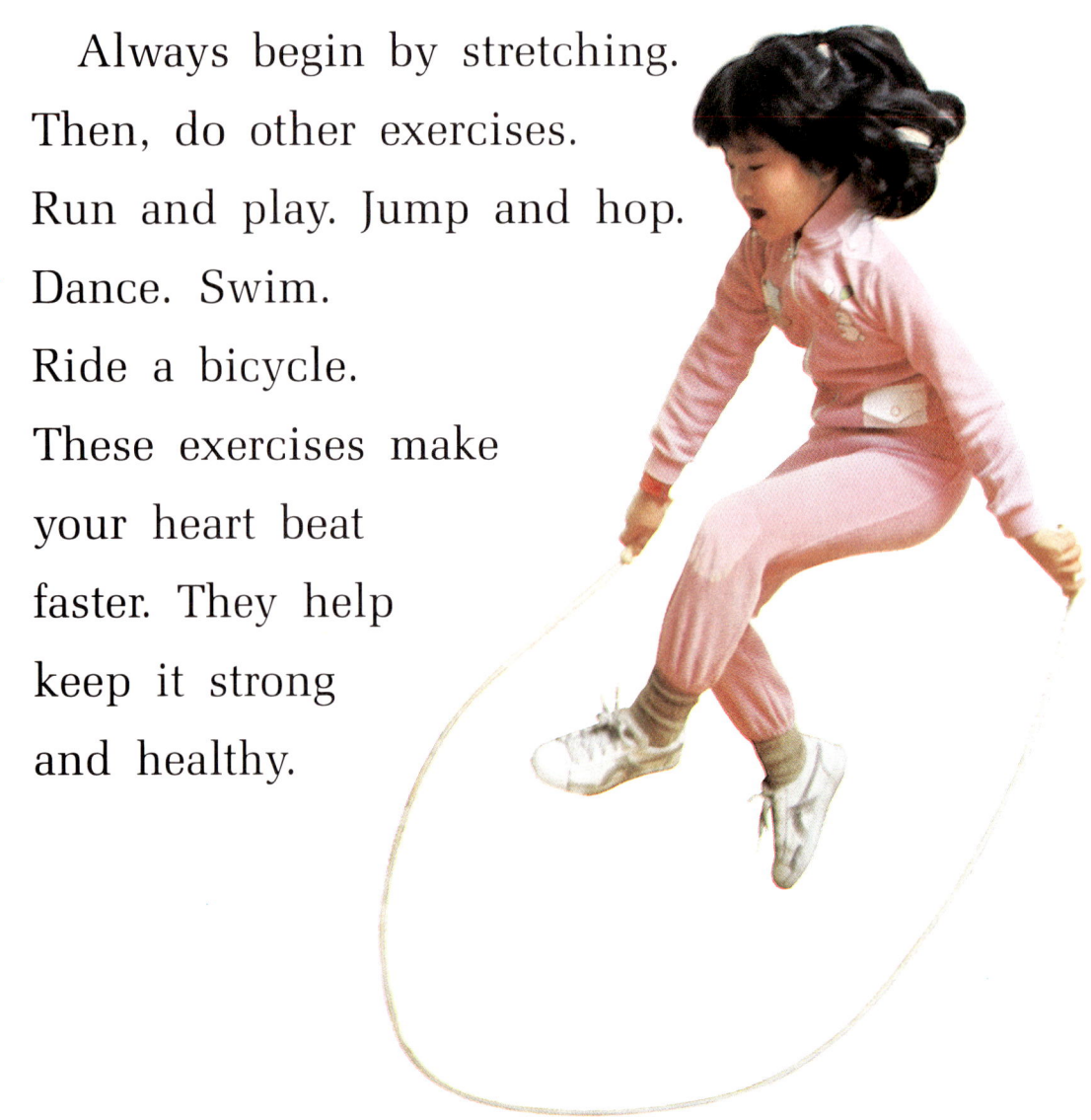

Always begin by stretching. Then, do other exercises. Run and play. Jump and hop. Dance. Swim. Ride a bicycle. These exercises make your heart beat faster. They help keep it strong and healthy.

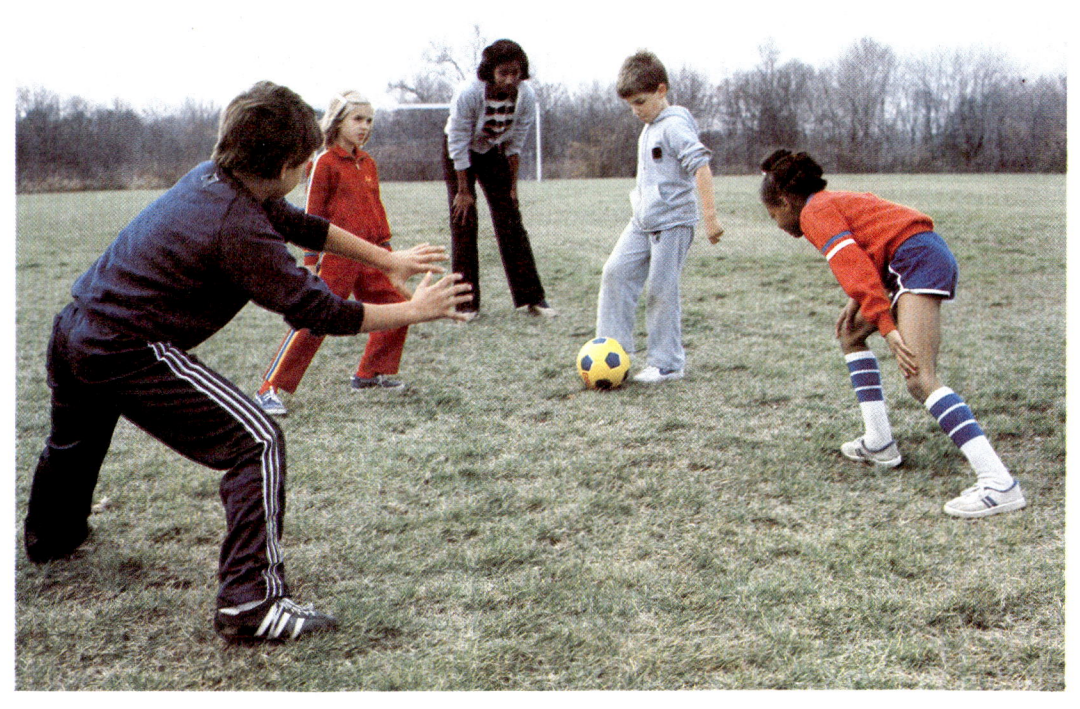

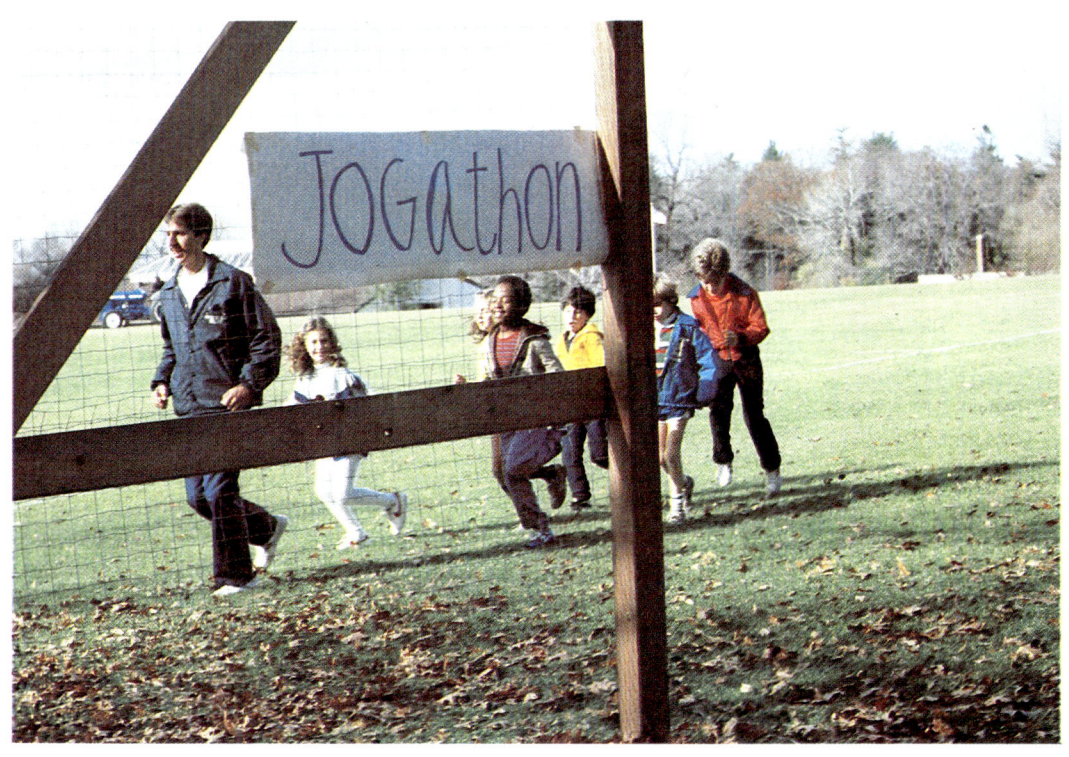

Cooling Down

Do not stop exercising all at once. Give your body a chance to cool down slowly. Do some stretching exercises. Do some other easy exercises. Do each one slowly. Do each for only a short time. Then, stop and let your body rest. Take a deep breath. Let it out.

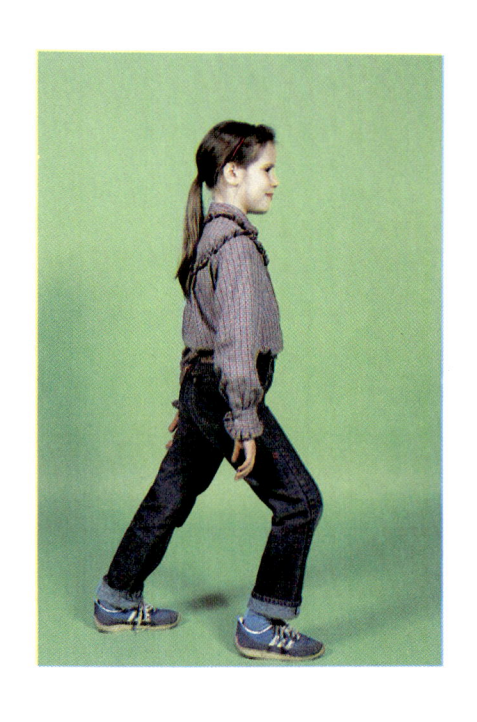

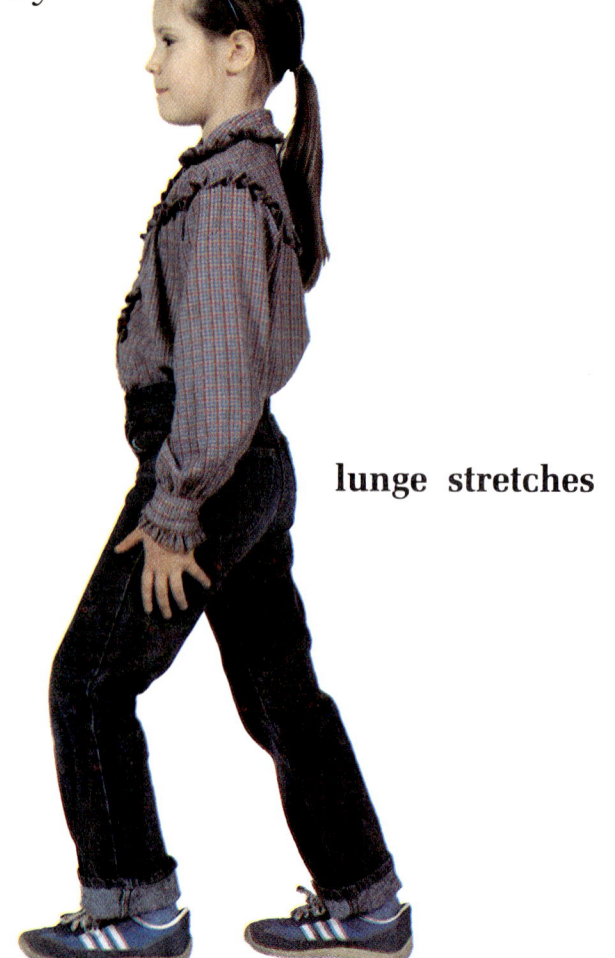

lunge stretches

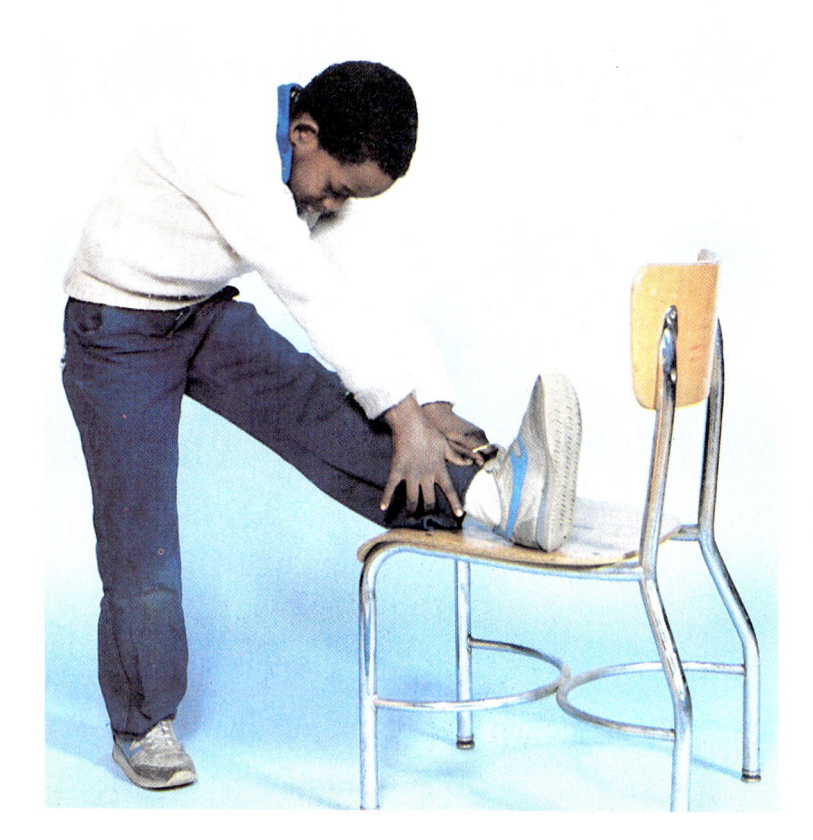

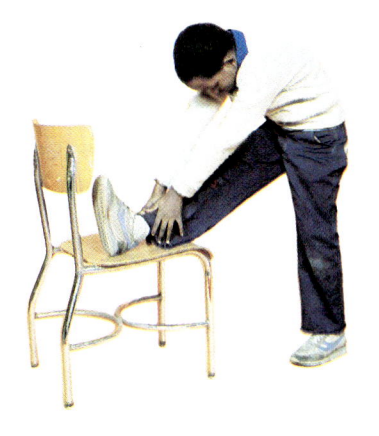

leg stretches

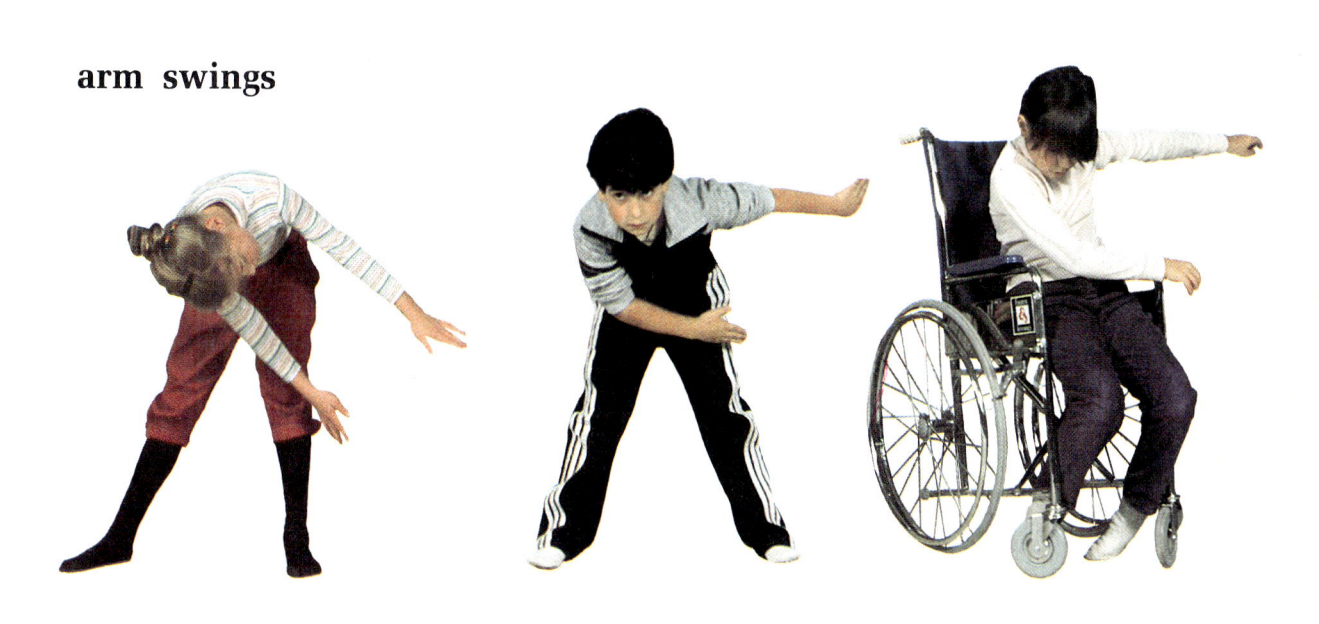

arm swings

Reviewing the HEALTH WORDS

The health words in the list are from the first page of each chapter. After each word is its meaning. Then, the word is used in a sentence. The number in dark print tells where to find the word in the book.

A

accident, something that happens that is not planned for. Kris had an accident on his bike and got hurt. **142**

afraid, feeling scared. Joel was afraid of the snake. **4**

B

body, all the parts that make up a person. Brad knows that exercise helps keep his body healthy. **26**

brush, to clean teeth with a toothbrush. Pat tries to brush her teeth after eating. **62**

C

caffeine, a drug that can be found in coffee, tea, and cola. Michael chose a drink without caffeine. **124**

cereal, a kind of food made from oats, wheat, rice, or other grains. Doreen ate bran cereal for breakfast. **54**

check-up, when a doctor or dentist looks at your body or teeth to see if they are healthy. Jerry had a check-up once a year. **94**

cough, something often done when someone has a cold. Jonathan covered his mouth when he started to cough. **74**

crossing guard, a person trained to help people cross a street safely. Donny waited until the crossing guard said it was safe to cross. **132**

crosswalk, the part of a street that is marked off for people to use when crossing. Jay looks for a crosswalk when he wants to cross a street. **132**

crown, the part of a tooth you can see. Mark brushed the crown of each of his teeth. **70**

D

decay, when a tooth has a cavity. Kim brushed her teeth often to help fight tooth decay. **72**

dentist, a person who is trained to take care of the teeth. The dentist showed Galia how to floss her teeth. **76**

diet, the food a person eats and drinks. Brenda's diet is made of food from the four food groups. **58**

disease, an illness. Some medicines can help fight disease. **110**

doctor, a person trained to give health care. The doctor gives David a check-up once a year. **94**

drug, something that can make a change in the body. A drug that helps the body is called a medicine. **114**

E

electricity, the power that makes lights, radios, and many other things work. Radios run on electricity. **156**

energy, the power to do things. Eating healthful food gives Gail <u>energy</u>. **36**

environment, surroundings. Everyone should help take care of the <u>environment</u>. **154**

F

family members, brothers, sisters, parents, grandparents, and other people who are related to one another. All the <u>family members</u> got together for a party once a year. **14**

features, the parts of the face and body that make up how a person looks. Jane and her parents have some of the same <u>features</u>. **24**

feelings, happy, sad, and afraid are kinds of feelings. Gary's <u>feelings</u> about the game changed many times. **4**

first aid, a kind of help given in an emergency. George needed <u>first aid</u> after the accident. **146**

floss, to use a special kind of string to clean between the teeth. The dentist told Greta to <u>floss</u> before bedtime. **70**

food groups, the four basic groups of food. Hector ate foods from the four <u>food groups</u> every day. **46**

friends, people who like one another. Anna and her <u>friends</u> have fun. **12**

front teeth, the teeth used to bite into food. Alex bit into the apple with his <u>front teeth</u>. **56**

fruit, part of a flowering plant you can eat. Jan's favorite <u>fruit</u> is apples. **48**

G

germs, tiny, living things. Some <u>germs</u> can make people ill. **74**

grains, seeds that come from wheat, rice, and some other kinds of plants. Justin eats foods made from <u>grains</u> every day. **55**

growing, getting bigger. Carol is <u>growing</u> out of her clothes. **26**

H

happy, feeling pleased about something. Mara was <u>happy</u> to see her mother. **4**

heart, the part of the body that pumps blood. When Paul exercises, his <u>heart</u> beats faster. **26**

L

lifeguard, a person trained to protect the safety of swimmers. The <u>lifeguard</u> taught Ricky how to swim. **142**

litter, trash left lying around. Patty picked up a piece of <u>litter</u> and put it in the trash can. **166**

love, to have a special feeling for someone. Steve and Merril kiss their grandmother because they <u>love</u> her. **13**

lungs, the parts of the body that are used for breathing. The doctor listened to Frank's <u>lungs</u> during his check-up. **26**

M

meat, a kind of food. Lisa had three slices of <u>meat</u> for supper. **50**

medicine, a drug used to help fight illness. Dr. Li gave Jo some <u>medicine</u>. **110**

milk, a food that comes from cows and some other animals. Marsha drank <u>milk</u> every day. **52**

molars, the teeth used for chewing food. Julio had four <u>molars</u> in the back of his mouth. **68**

181

muscles, parts of the body that help the body move. Lee could jump high because she had strong leg muscles. **26**

N

natural resources, coal, oil, and some other things found in and on the earth. Al showered quickly to save water, one of our natural resources. **156**

nicotine, a drug found in tobacco smoke. The nicotine in tobacco smoke harmed Mr. Benson's heart and lungs. **122**

nurse, a person trained to give some kinds of health care. The nurse weighed Rita and measured her height. **102**

P

permanent teeth, the second set of teeth that grows in. Mrs. Malko has all her permanent teeth. **68**

pharmacist, a person trained to prepare medicine. The pharmacist called Marcello's doctor about the medicine. **120**

poison, something that is harmful if taken into the body. Mr. Chen put the poison on a high shelf. **118**

pollution, something that harms the environment. Noise is a kind of pollution. **164**

primary teeth, the first set of teeth that grows in. Lil has 20 primary teeth. **68**

S

sad, feeling unhappy. Jack was sad when his friend moved away. **4**

safety, not being in danger. Terry cares about her safety. **132**

seatbelt, strap in a car that helps hold a person in the seat. Mat kept his seatbelt buckled for the whole car trip. **138**

senses, hearing, sight, touch, taste, and smell are the senes. Ellen used all her senses to learn about the new food. **28**

share, to use something with someone else. Rob and Bill often share their toys. **14**

sneeze, something often done when someone has a cold. Brenda covered her nose and mouth as she started to sneeze. **88**

T

tar, one of the harmful things in tobacco smoke. Tar can harm anyone who breathes tobacco smoke. **122**

thoughtful, being kind. Sandy has many friends because she is thoughtful. **12**

traffic, the cars, buses, and trucks moving along a street. When the traffic stopped, Pablo crossed the street. **132**

V

vegetable, a plant used as food. Patty had a vegetable with her supper. **48**

vision, being able to see. Gloria liked wearing her glasses because they helped her vision. **96**

W

water, something that everyone needs to live. Marjorie drinks a lot of water every day. **158**

Index

A

Accidents, prevention of, 142-147, 144 (*Illus.*), 146 (*Illus.*),149-151
Addis, William, 74
Angry (feelings), 4, 6, 8
Animals, safety around, 130, 140-141, 140-141 (*Illus.*), 148, 148 (*Illus.*), 151
Art, 162-163, 162 (*Illus.*)
Asking, for help with medicine, 102, 112, 115, 118-120, 119 (*Illus.*), 127-128

B

Beans (meat group), 50, 50 (*Illus.*), 65
Bicycle safety, 134-137, 134-135 (*Illus.*), 150
Body, 10, 10 (*Illus.*), 26, 26 (*Illus.*), 27 (*Illus.*), 31, 35-36, 38, 41, 41 (*Illus.*), 42, 44, 50-51, 53, 55-58, 60, 84, 90, 94, 94 (*Illus.*), 100-102, 100-102 (*Illus.*), 105, 107, 108-110, 118, 123, 123 (*Illus.*), 127, 129 (See also **Ears, Eyes.**)
  bones, 26, 52, 74, 102, 114
  heart, 26, 41 (*Illus.*), 100, 100 (*Illus.*), 114, 122-124
  lungs, 26, 41 (*Illus.*), 100, 101 (*Illus.*), 122-123, 123 (*Illus.*)
  muscles, 26, 41 (*Illus.*), 50, 102, 174
  nose, 41, 90
Bones (See under **Body.**)

Bread (bread and cereal group), 46, 54, 55 (*Illus.*), 65
Breakfast, 55, 57, 59 (*Illus.*)
Breathing, 100, 122-123, 123 (*Illus.*), 127
Brushing
  hair, 39 (*Illus.*), 43
  teeth, 38, 38 (*Illus.*), 72-74, 72 (*Illus.*), 82-83
Buses (See under **Safety.**)

C

Caffeine, 124-125, 124-125 (*Illus.*), 127, 129
  in cocoa, 124, 124 (*Illus.*)
  in cola drinks, 124, 124 (*Illus.*), 126, 126 (*Illus.*)
Cars (See under **Safety.**)
Cereal (bread and cereal group), 46, 54-55, 54-55 (*Illus.*)
Check-up, 66, 81, 82, 94, 94-96 (*Illus.*), 100-101, 100-101 (*Illus.*)
  dental, 66, 81, 82
  medical, 94, 94-96 (*Illus.*), 100-101, 100-101(*Illus.*)
Cheese (milk group), 52-53 (*Illus.*), 65
Chicken (meat group), 50
Cleanliness, 38, 38 (*Illus.*)
Cold (illness) 92-93, 92-93 (*Illus.*), 99, 107
Color blindness, 32, 32 (*Illus.*)
Cooling-down exercises, 178-179, 178-179 (*Illus.*)
Coughing, 88, 88 (*Illus.*)

Crossing the street, 31, 129-134, 132-133 (*Illus.*), 137, 150-151
  corners, 132, 132 (*Illus.*), 137 (*Illus.*), 151
  crosswalk, 132, 132 (*Illus.*), 133 (*Illus.*), 137 (*Illus.*)
Crown (See under **Teeth.**)

D

Decay, tooth, 72, 76, 83
Dentist, 76-77, 76-77 (*Illus.*), 81-83
Diet, 58, 63-64
Dinner, 18
Directions, following, 112-113
Disease, 110-111, 115, 115 (*Illus.*), 129
Doctor, 85 (*Illus.*), 94-96, 95 (*Illus.*), 100-102, 101 (*Illus.*), 105, 107, 116, 120, 120 (*Illus.*), 174
Drugs, 108-117, 128-129
Dunlop, John, 136

E

Ears, 30-31, 30-31 (*Illus.*), 94, 94 (*Illus.*), 164-165, 172-173
  protection of, 164-165, 172-173
Eating, for good health, 36-37, 37 (*Illus.*), 43, 44-66, 72
  meals, 36, 36 (*Illus.*), 46 (*Illus.*), 58-59, 58-59 (*Illus.*), 62-63, 62 (*Illus.*), 72
  safely, 118, 128
  servings, 50-51, 54
  snacks, 60-61, 63, 65

183

Eggs (meat group), 50, 65
Electricity (See under **Saving**.)
Energy, 36, 36 (*Illus.*), 44, 54, 58, 63 (See also under **Saving**.)
Environment, caring for, 152, 152-153 (*Illus.*), 154-155, 154-155 (*Illus.*), 164, 168-169, 168-169 (*Illus.*), 171, 173
Exercise, 36, 36 (*Illus.*), 174-179, 174-179 (*Illus.*)
Eyes, 24, 24 (*Illus.*), 30-31, 30-31 (*Illus.*), 48, 94
  eyeglasses, 96-97, 97 (*Illus.*), 105
  testing, 95 (*Illus.*), 96-97, 96 (*Illus.*)

F
Family, 14-18, 14-18 (*Illus.*), 24-25, 25 (*Illus.*), 46, 90, 96, 102, 120, 149, 168, 168 (*Illus.*), 171
Feelings, 2, 3 (*Illus.*), 4-9, 5 (*Illus.*), 7 (*Illus.*), 8 (*Illus.*), 10-12, 10-12 (*Illus.*), 13 (*Illus.*), 19
  feeling good, 12, 14, 38, 78, 166, 174
  showing feelings, 3, 8-11, 8 (*Illus.*), 10-11 (*Illus.*), 13 (*Illus.*), 19
First aid, 146, 147 (*Illus.*), 151
Fish (meat group), 50
Flossing, 72-73, 73 (*Illus.*), 75, 75 (*Illus.*), 77 (*Illus.*), 80
Food, 28, 37 (*Illus.*), 44, 45-46 (*Illus.*), 47-65, 47-64 (*Illus.*), 70, 72, 89, 89 (*Illus.*), 108, 118-119, 118 (*Illus.*), 124-125, 124-125 (*Illus.*), 127 (See also **Eating**.)
  groups, 45 (*Illus.*), 46, 48-58, 48-58 (*Illus.*), 60, 64-65
Fruit (fruit and vegetable group), 46, 48-49, 48-49 (*Illus.*), 65

G
Germs, protection from, 72, 86-89, 86-88 (*Illus.*), 92, 92 (*Illus.*), 99, 105-107, 105 (*Illus.*), 110-111, 146
  tissue, use of, 92, 92 (*Illus.*), 107
Glasses, eye (See under **Eyes**.)
Grain (bread and cereal group), 54-55, 54-55 (*Illus.*)
Growing up, 22, 22 (*Illus.*)
Growth, physical, 22, 22 (*Illus.*), 23 (*Illus.*), 26-30, 26-27 (*Illus.*), 33-40, 33-37 (*Illus.*), 42-44, 50, 52, 58, 63, 65, 76, 94
Gums (See under **Teeth**.)

H
Habits, for good health, 36-37, 36-37 (*Illus.*), 38 (*Illus.*), 39, 39 (*Illus.*), 41-43
  for safety, 144-145, 150
Happy (feelings), 4, 4 (*Illus.*), 6, 7
Health, 17, 36-37, 37-38 (*Illus.*), 39, 39 (*Illus.*), 41-43, 48-50, 52, 84-107, 85 (*Illus.*), 94 (*Illus.*), 116 (See also **Resting, Staying well**.)
  eating for good health, see under **Eating**.
  habits for good health, see under **Habits**.
Hearing, 28, 28 (*Illus.*), 164-165, 164 (*Illus.*), 171-172
Heart (See under **Body**.)
Height, 24, 94
Home, 16, 18-19, 92-93, 144, 149, 149 (*Illus.*), 155 (*Illus.*), 163, 168-169, 168-169 (*Illus.*), 171-173
  helping care for, 16, 18-19, 155 (*Illus.*), 168-169, 168-169 (*Illus.*), 171, 173
  safety in, 144, 149, 149 (*Illus.*)

I
Illness, 86, 90, 90-92 (*Illus.*), 108, 118
Injury, 66, 79, 81, 129, 146, 174

J
Juice, 92, 92 (*Illus.*), 99 (*Illus.*), 107
Junk, use in art, 162, 162 (*Illus.*), 163 (*Illus.*)

K
Krill, 56, 56 (*Illus.*)

L
Labels, reading, 109 (*Illus.*), 112-113, 112-113 (*Illus.*), 115, 115 (*Illus.*), 118, 128-129
Learning, 22, 26-28, 40, 40 (*Illus.*), 43, 63, 77, 84, 94-95, 100-101, 107-108, 109 (*Illus.*), 113-114, 120 (*Illus.*), 128-129, 134
Litter, 166, 166 (*Illus.*), 173

Loving, 8 (*Illus.*), 14-15, 14-15 (*Illus.*)
Lunch, 56, 59 (*Illus.*)
Lungs (See under **Body.**)

M
Marceau, Marcel, 10, 10 (*Illus.*)
Meals (See under **Eating.**)
Meat (meat group), 46, 46 (*Illus.*), 50-51, 50-51 (*Illus.*), 56, 56 (*Illus.*), 65
Medicine, 109 (*Illus.*), 110-121, 110-118 (*Illus.*), 120-121 (*Illus.*), 127-129 (See also **Asking, Labels.**)
Mexico, 40
Milk (milk group), 46, 52-53, 52-53 (*Illus.*), 65
Mime, 10
Molar, 68-69, 68 (*Illus.*)
Muscles (See under **Body.**)

N
Natural resources, 156, 158, 173 (See also under **Saving.**)
Needs
 energy, 36
 help, 91, 96
 meat, 50, 50 (*Illus.*), 51 (*Illus.*)
 medicine, 112, 120
 milk, 52
 teeth, 78
Nicotine, 122, 129
Noise, 140, 164, 164 (*Illus.*), 171-173
Nose (See under **Body.**)
Nurse, 85 (*Illus.*), 90-102, 102 (*Illus.*), 110 (*Illus.*), 116, 120
Nuts (meat group), 50

O
Oats (bread and cereal group), 54-55

P
Paper, 158 (*Illus.*) (See also under **Saving.**)
Permanent teeth, 68-69, 68-69 (*Illus.*), 75-76
Pharmacist, 120, 121 (*Illus.*), 129
Playing safely, 142, 142 (*Illus.*)
Poison, 118-119, 118 (*Illus.*)
Pollution, 164, 164 (*Illus.*), 166, 171-173
Primary teeth, 68-69, 68-69 (*Illus.*), 75, 83
Protection
 of body, 110, 115, 129, 174
 of environment, 152-155, 152-155 (*Illus.*), 164, 164 (*Illus.*), 168, 168 (*Illus.*), 171, 173
 of hearing, 164-165, 164 (*Illus.*), 171-172
 of teeth, 66, 78-79, 78-79 (*Illus.*), 81

R
Reading labels (See under **Labels.**)
Resting, for good health, 36, 92
Rice (bread and cereal group), 54-55, 65
Riding (See **Bicycle safety;** see also under **Safety.**)
Root (See under **Teeth.**)
Rules for safety (See under **Safety.**)
Running games, 142, 149, 151

S
Sadness, 4, 6, 8
Safety, 30-32, 30-32 (*Illus.*), 34, 78, 78 (*Illus.*), 82, 127, 129-151, 130-149 (*Illus.*), 152 (See also **Bicycle safety, Crossing the street, First aid, Labels, Playing safely, Traffic and safety;** see under **Home.**)
 and the environment, 142-143, 154 (*Illus.*)
 riding in buses, 130, 138-139, 138 (*Illus.*), 149, 151
 riding in cars, 130, 132, 134, 137 (*Illus.*), 138-139
 rules for, 132, 134-135, 137-139, 143, 149-150, 149 (*Illus.*)
Saving
 electricity, 157 (*Illus.*), 173
 energy, 156-157, 157 (*Illus.*), 172
 natural resources, 160-161, 160-161 (*Illus.*), 163, 163 (*Illus.*), 170-171, 170-171 (*Illus.*)
 paper, 158-159, 163, 172
 water, 158-159, 159 (*Illus.*)
Scrape, treating a, 102, 103 (*Illus.*), 146, 147 (*Illus.*), 151
Seatbelt, 138, 139 (*Illus.*)
Seeing, 28, 28 (*Illus.*), 32, 32 (*Illus.*), 96, 98, 98 (*Illus.*), 104
Senses, physical, 28-31, 28 (*Illus.*), 33-35, 33-35 (*Illus.*), 40, 40 (*Illus.*), 42, 43 (See also **Seeing.**)
 smell, 28, 28 (*Illus.*), 34-35, 34-35 (*Illus.*), 41, 41 (*Illus.*), 43

taste, 28, 28 (*Illus.*), 118-119
touch, 28, 28 (*Illus.*), 34-35, 34-35 (*Illus.*)
Servings (See under **Eating**.)
Sharing with others, 12, 14, 16, 88-89, 88-89 (*Illus.*), 99, 173
Smell, sense of (See **Senses**.)
Smoke, 34, 127
Smoking, 122-123, 122-123 (*Illus.*), 127-128
Snacks (See under **Eating**.)
Sneezing, 88, 88 (*Illus.*)
Staying well, 44, 58, 65, 84, 93, 154, 156-158, 157 (*Illus.*), 160
Street, see **Crossing the street.**
Stretching exercises, 174-175 (*Illus.*)
Supper, 58 (*Illus.*)
Sweets, in diet, 66, 72

T
Tall (See **Height**.)
Taste (See under **Senses**.)
Teeth, 38, 38 (*Illus.*), 48, 52, 66-83, 66-81 (*Illus.*)
  cleaning and care of, 38, 38 (*Illus.*), 48, 52, 66, 66 (*Illus.*), 69, 70-83, 70-81 (*Illus.*), (See also **Permanent teeth, Primary teeth**.)
  crown, 70-71, 70 (*Illus.*), 81, 81 (*Illus.*), 83
  gums, 48, 69 (*Illus.*), 70-71, 70 (*Illus.*), 76, 81, 83
  root, 70-71, 70 (*Illus.*), 81
Tinguely, Jean, 162, 162 (*Illus.*)

Tires, bicycle, 136, 136 (*Illus.*)
Tissue (See under **Germs**.)
Tobacco smoke, 122-123, 122-123 (*Illus.*), 129
Tooth, parts of, 81, 81 (*Illus.*) (See also under **Teeth**.)
Toothbrush, 74, 74-75 (*Illus.*), 80
Tooth decay, 72, 76, 83
Touch (See under **Senses**.)
Traffic and safety, 132, 132 (*Illus.*), 134, 135 (*Illus.*), 137 (*Illus.*)
  lights, 32 (*Illus.*), 132, 132 (*Illus.*), 135 (*Illus.*)
Trash, 166, 166 (*Illus.*), 173
  trash can, 166, 166 (*Illus.*)
Trees, 158, 172-173
Tricycle, 136, 136 (*Illus.*)
Turkey (meat group), 50

V
Vegetables (fruit and vegetable group), 46, 48-49, 48-49 (*Illus.*), 63, 65
Vision (See **Seeing**.)

W
Warming-up exercises, 175 (*Illus.*)
Water, 11, 58, 78, 86, 92, 142, 143 (*Illus.*), 150, 158-159, 159 (*Illus.*) (See also under **Saving**.)
  fountain, 78, 78 (*Illus.*)
Wheat (bread and cereal group), 54-55
Wheel, 136, 136 (*Illus.*)